Adult-Gerontology Acute Care Nurse Practitioner Exam Practice Questions

NP Practice Tests & Exam Review for the
Nurse Practitioner Exam

Dear Future Exam Success Story:

First of all, **THANK YOU** for purchasing Mometrix study materials!

Second, congratulations! You are one of the few determined test-takers who are committed to doing whatever it takes to excel on your exam. **You have come to the right place.** We developed these practice tests with one goal in mind: to deliver you the best possible approximation of the questions you will see on test day.

Standardized testing is one of the biggest obstacles on your road to success, which only increases the importance of doing well in the high-pressure, high-stakes environment of test day. Your results on this test could have a significant impact on your future, and these practice tests will give you the repetitions you need to build your familiarity and confidence with the test content and format to help you achieve your full potential on test day.

Your success is our success

We would love to hear from you! If you would like to share the story of your exam success or if you have any questions or comments in regard to our products, please contact us at **800-673-8175** or **support@mometrix.com**.

Thanks again for your business and we wish you continued success!

Sincerely,
The Mometrix Test Preparation Team

TABLE OF CONTENTS

Practice Test #1

1. Patients with severe nausea and vomiting not associated with pain are most at risk for:
    a. hyperkalemia.
    b. hypokalemia.
    c. hypercalcemia.
    d. hypocalcemia.

2. If a 54-year-old patient is to begin a short-term sleeping aid, such as eszopiclone (Lunesta), for persistent insomnia, the adult-gerontology acute care nurse practitioner (AGACNP) should document warning the patient to avoid:
    a. eating or drinking milk products.
    b. exercising and climbing stairs.
    c. operating heavy machinery and driving.
    d. taking vitamins or minerals.

3. A 69-year-old patient received an accidental overdose of heparin. Which of the following allergies places the patient at risk for anaphylactic reaction to protamine, the heparin antagonist?
    a. Milk products.
    b. Tree nuts.
    c. Soy.
    d. Fish products.

4. Pharmacokinetics refers to the:
    a. effects the body has on a drug.
    b. effects a drug has on the body.
    c. way drugs interact with each other.
    d. study of how drugs affect the body.

5. A 26-year-old male patient comes to the emergency department complaining of purulent urethral discharge and urinary frequency and burning with increasing severity over 3 days. During the assessment, the patient admits to an encounter with a prostitute 7 days earlier. The Gram stain shows the presence of Gram-negative bacteria, but the culture and sensitivity results will be delayed. The appropriate treatment approach is:
    a. waiting for culture and sensitivity results before prescribing treatment.
    b. prescribing cefatrizine (intramuscularly [IM]) and azithromycin (by mouth [po]) in single doses.
    c. prescribing ciprofloxacin (po) in a single dose.
    d. prescribing cefatrizine (intravenously [IV]) daily until symptoms subside and then cefixime daily for one week.

6. Abnormal pulsus paradoxus is characterized by:
    a. systolic blood pressure ≤5 mm Hg higher during inhalation than exhalation.
    b. systolic blood pressure ≤5 mm Hg lower during inhalation than exhalation
    c. systolic blood pressure >10 mm Hg higher during inhalation than exhalation.
    d. systolic blood pressure >10 mm Hg lower during inhalation than exhalation.

7. Using the RIFLE criteria for classifying increasing renal failure, a 62-year-old patient with an increase of serum creatinine of 200% or a decrease in glomerular filtration rate of >50% with urine output of <0.5 mL/kg/hr over 12 hours is classified as:

    a. loss.
    b. risk.
    c. injury.
    d. failure.

8. Which of the following is an example of a dementia-associated condition resulting from an environmental cause?

    a. AIDS.
    b. Parkinson's disease.
    c. Huntington's disease.
    d. Alzheimer's disease.

9. On assessment, the AGACNP observes that an 82-year-old patient has bruises on both forearms and her face. The patient admits that her daughter sometimes gets angry and hits her but "feels terrible afterward." The patient begs the AGACNP to "forget about it." The AGACNP should:

    a. take no action per patient request.
    b. report the abuse to the appropriate authorities.
    c. warn the daughter not to repeat the abuse.
    d. refer the patient and daughter for counseling.

10. A 20-year-old patient who recently returned from a trip to Mexico has developed watery diarrhea with severe dehydration. The patient exhibits confusion, hypotension, and tachypnea, and the AGACNP suspects metabolic acidosis. The critical value for serum pH with metabolic acidosis is:

    a. 7.40.
    b. 7.0.
    c. >7.60.
    d. <7.20.

11. What is a good strategy for helping an elderly client overcome feelings of low self-esteem related to chronic illness and loss of autonomy?

    a. Praise the client constantly for any activities.
    b. Tell the client she has no reason to feel so depressed.
    c. Provide opportunities for the client to make decisions.
    d. Encourage the patient to focus on positive factors.

12. A 70-year-old male patient is admitted with right-sided heart failure. Findings that are consistent with right-side heart failure include:

    a. paroxysmal nocturnal dyspnea.
    b. increased jugular venous pressure.
    c. pulmonary venous congestion.
    d. orthopnea.

13. A visitor stops the AGACNP and asks, "Could you tell me what is wrong with the patient across the hall from my husband? He seems so agitated." The response that complies with the Health Insurance Portability and Accountability Act (HIPAA) is:

    a. "The law doesn't allow me to give out any information about patients in order to protect their privacy and safety."
    b. "His wife is in the lounge. You can go ask her."
    c. "Why are you asking?"
    d. "He has kidney disease, like your husband."

14. A 76-year-old female dresses in youthful styles, acts in a girlish manner, and states repeatedly that she hates getting older. According to Erikson's psychosocial development model, which stage is she experiencing?

    a. Identity vs. role confusion.
    b. Industry vs. inferiority.
    c. Ego integrity vs. despair.
    d. Generativity vs. stagnation.

15. A patient refuses to participate in physical therapy, stating, "I don't want to do this!" When using the SOAP format, this statement would be documented in:

    a. subjective.
    b. objective
    c. assessment.
    d. plan.

16. A 52-year-old patient with heart disease is having difficulty with smoking cessation. The AGACNP should advise the patient that the most effective method of reducing the temptation to smoke is to:

    a. wait out the urge.
    b. substitute something else for cigarettes.
    c. practice relaxation exercises.
    d. avoid triggers.

17. When determining the burden of proof for acts of negligence, risk management would classify willfully providing inadequate care while disregarding the safety and security of another as:

    a. negligent conduct.
    b. gross negligence.
    c. contributory negligence.
    d. comparative negligence.

18. When the AGACNP delegates a task to another healthcare provider, the most important consideration when choosing the right person is:

    a. availability.
    b. reliability.
    c. education/skills.
    d. years of experience.

19. Which of the following tests is most accurate for determining acute changes in nutritional status to monitor dietary compliance for a 15-year-old patient with anorexia?

    a. Transferrin.
    b. Total protein.
    c. Albumin.
    d. Prealbumin.

20. An 80-year-old woman has a sudden onset of right-sided paresis, short-term memory loss, depression, right visual field defect, and mild expressive aphasia, indicating a possible stroke. The most likely part of the brain affected is the:

    a. right hemisphere.
    b. left hemisphere.
    c. brain stem.
    d. cerebellum.

21. When assessing a patient with a history of alcohol abuse, the laboratory study that is especially important to include is:

    a. liver function tests.
    b. pulmonary function tests.
    c. renal function tests.
    d. thyroid function tests.

22. If a 15-year-old female patient reports that an adult touched her "private parts" against her wishes, the most appropriate statement or question by the AGACNP is:

    a. "That must have been terrifying for you to experience."
    b. "Did you scream or fight back in any way?"
    c. "Why do you think that happened to you?"
    d. "What specific part of your body do you mean when you say 'private parts'?"

23. For quality/performance improvement, the best tool to determine methods to streamline processes is:

    a. root cause analysis.
    b. the tracer methodology.
    c. family survey.
    d. staff survey.

24. The greatest risk factor for the development of methicillin-resistant *Staphylococcus aureus* (MRSA) pneumonia is:

    a. inadequate turning, coughing, and deep-breathing.
    b. hospitalization on a medical-surgical floor.
    c. exposure to people with a cough.
    d. intubation and ventilation.

25. Distribution of drugs is often impaired in gerontological patients because of:

    a. changes in body water volume.
    b. increased gastric pH.
    c. changes in hepatic volume.
    d. reduced renal blood flow.

26. If a patient is diagnosed with Parkinson's disease but symptoms are very mild, levodopa is often withheld until symptoms worsen because:

    a. the treatment regimen is difficult to manage.
    b. the drug is ineffective for mild symptoms.
    c. the drug's effectiveness decreases over time.
    d. the side effects are severe.

27. Prior to a nasogastric tube feeding, a pH check of aspirant reveals a pH of 8. Which of the following does this most likely indicate?

    a. The tube tip is in the stomach.
    b. The tube tip in in the respiratory system.
    c. The tube tip is in the small intestine.
    d. The tube tip is in the esophagus.

28. A patient being treated for a gastric ulcer has been stable on medications. Which of the following indicates a possible emergent situation?

    a. Inability to sleep well and generalized anxiety.
    b. Periodic epigastric pain (heartburn) relieved by medications.
    c. Nausea after taking prescribed antibiotics.
    d. Increasing back and epigastric pain unrelieved by medications.

29. When measuring the ankle-brachial index (ABI), how far above the last sound heard on Doppler ultrasound should the blood pressure cuff be pumped?

    a. 5 mm Hg.
    b. 10 mm Hg.
    c. 20 mm Hg.
    d. 30 mm Hg.

30. Which of the following is an indication that a patient with diabetes has developed Charcot foot?

    a. Rocker-bottom-shaped foot.
    b. Foot ulcerations.
    c. Peripheral neuropathic pain.
    d. Lack of pain sensation in the foot.

31. A 60-year-old male patient has mild prostatic hypertrophy with no urinary retention. The treatment of choice is likely:

    a. transurethral resection of the prostate (TURP).
    b. watch and wait.
    c. 5-alpha-reductase inhibitor.
    d. alpha-blocker.

32. In evidence-based research, what does persistent erratic findings in tracking and trending suggest?

    a. Changes in patient population requiring changes in processes of care.
    b. Errors in statistical analysis of processes of care.
    c. Normal day-to-day variations in processes of care.
    d. Processes of care are not consistent or are inadequate.

33. Which type of diet is usually recommended for those with chronic pancreatitis?

    a. Low protein.
    b. Low carbohydrate.
    c. Low fat.
    d. Gluten free.

34. A patient receiving total parenteral nutrition (TPN) for inflammatory bowel disease should be monitored every 6 hours for which of the following?

    a. Hemoglobin and hematocrit.
    b. Blood glucose level.
    c. Blood, urea, nitrogen (BUN).
    d. Electrolytes.

35. A 28-year-old patient with three young children has ovarian cancer and is to be discharged to her home with fentanyl transdermal patches for pain control. When teaching the patient about the use of the patches, the AGACNP should stress that discarded patches:

    a. must be immediately flushed down the toilet.
    b. can be discarded into any wastebasket.
    c. should be cut into small pieces before discarding.
    d. can be discarded in any manner because they are harmless.

36. A 26-year-old patient presents with a rapidly developing sore throat that is severely painful, especially when attempting to swallow. The patient is sitting in the tripod position with her mouth open, and she is drooling. These signs and symptoms are characteristic of:

    a. strep throat.
    b. epiglottitis.
    c. tonsillitis
    d. peritonsillar abscess.

37. The most common cause of distributive shock is:

    a. acute adrenal insufficiency.
    b. vasodilator drugs.
    c. anaphylaxis.
    d. sepsis.

38. If the AGACNP is conducting clinical research and intends to select participants that will be able to provide a particular perspective related to the research question, this type of sampling is referred to as:

    a. purposeful.
    b. nominated.
    c. convenience.
    d. theoretical.

39. A patient was recently divorced and makes the following negative statement: "I can't manage on my own." Which of the following is the most therapeutic response in helping the patient cope with this stressful situation?

    a. "I understand how upset you are."
    b. "Of course you can! You're a strong person."
    c. "Can you think of something positive about being on your own?"
    d. "You have a lot of possibilities now that you are on your own."

40. A 49-year-old male complains of severe chest pain radiating to the left shoulder and arm. The vital signs are as follows: blood pressure (BP), 152/92; pulse (P), 96; respirations (R), 20. Oxygen saturation is 94%, and temperature is 38°C (100.4°F). The patient is nauseated, and his skin is clammy. The electrocardiogram (ECG) shows anterior ST-segment elevation myocardial infarction (STEMI). The treatment priority should include:

    a. beta blocker.
    b. ACE inhibitor.
    c. oxygen.
    d. acetylsalicylic acid (ASA) and nitrates.

41. Which of the following is a realistic goal for the AGACNP to include in the care plan of a patient with diabetes mellitus?

    a. A1c <5%.
    b. A1c <7%.
    c. Preprandial glucose of 60 to 100 mg/dL.
    d. Postprandial glucose of <120 mg/dL.

42. If an adult patient with intermittent asthma begins wheezing and shows little improvement with an inhaled short-acting beta-2 agonist (SABA) such as albuterol, the next step in the treatment of choice is:

    a. inhaled long-acting beta-2 agonist (LABA).
    b. oral corticosteroid.
    c. low-dose inhaled corticosteroid (ICS).
    d. theophylline.

43. A patient being treated for endocarditis has developed sudden-onset hematuria. The AGACNP should suspect:

    a. renal embolization.
    b. urinary tract infection.
    c. drug reaction.
    d. bladder hemorrhage.

44. A 78-year-old patient with chronic obstructive pulmonary disease (COPD) hospitalized with acute respiratory distress syndrome (ARDS) has pronounced wheezing, fever (38.6°C [101.5°F]), and cough. Arterial blood gases are pH, 7.24; PaO_2, 49 mm Hg; and $PaCO_2$, 61 mm Hg. The AGACNP prescribes a steroid and a bronchodilator. The patient is alert and able to follow directions but remains unable to speak because of dyspnea. Which treatment is most appropriate to relieve respiratory distress?

    a. Oxygen therapy only.
    b. Intubation and assist/control (AC) ventilation.
    c. Intubation and synchronized intermittent mandatory ventilation (SIMV).
    d. Noninvasive ventilation (NIV).

45. The AGACNP works with a group of ethnically diverse staff members, but a number of conflicts have arisen because of different methods of communication and attitudes toward authority. The best solution is likely to:

    a. initiate a discussion about cultural differences.
    b. issue guidelines regarding effective communication.
    c. ignore the situation and give it time to resolve.
    d. seek outside assistance in conflict resolution.

46. If a patient is receiving methotrexate for maintenance treatment of Crohn's disease, which laboratory tests should be routinely monitored?

    a. Complete blood count (CBC) and renal function tests.
    b. CBC and sedimentation rate.
    c. CBC, renal function, and liver function tests.
    d. CBC and pancreatic enzymes.

47. If a 19-year-old female patient with sickle cell disease experienced an aplastic crisis with hemoglobin of 5.6 g/dL (56 mmol/L), she will likely receive transfusions of packed red blood cells until her hemoglobin reaches:

    a. 8 g/dL (80 mmol/L).
    b. 10 g/dL (100 mmol/L).
    c. 12 g/dL (120 mmol/L).
    d. 14 g/dL (140 mmol/L).

48. A patient who was the victim of a violent assault and rape is shaking and crying and appears terrified. Which of the following responses is most therapeutic at the initial encounter with the patient?

    a. "Why are you crying?"
    b. "I can see that you are still frightened."
    c. "What can I do to help you?"
    d. "You are safe now."

49. The AGACNP examines a patient's functional ability and notes that his gait is characterized by shuffling of the feet with periodic short rapid steps while the neck, trunk, and knees are flexed and the patient leaning forward, increasingly walking faster. The AGACNP should recognize this gait as being characteristic of:

    a. Parkinson's disease.
    b. cerebral palsy.
    c. hemiplegia.
    d. developmental dysplasia of the hip.

50. A 60-year-old patient's BP ranges from 140–159/90–99. This BP is classified as:

    a. normal.
    b. prehypertension.
    c. stage 1 hypertension.
    d. stage 2 hypertension.

51. An 86-year-old patient has developed blistering, painful lesions extending from the left side of her back around to the left side of her chest, indicating probable herpes zoster (shingles) infection. The most appropriate treatment is:

    a. corticosteroid (such as prednisone).
    b. antiviral (such as acyclovir).
    c. antibiotic (such as ampicillin).
    d. analgesia only.

52. A patient under end-of-life hospice care for stage 4 multiple myeloma has developed severe skeletal pain and is scheduled to undergo radiation therapy to reduce discomfort. How will this treatment affect hospice care?

    a. Hospice care must be discontinued.
    b. Hospice care is put on hold until treatment is finished and then resumed.
    c. Hospice care will continue without interruption.
    d. Hospice care may be continued if preauthorization is received.

53. Which of the following patients is most at risk for development of a chronic subdural hematoma 3 to 4 weeks after the initial injury?

    a. 18-year-old patient who developed a concussion from a football injury.
    b. 28-year-old patient who struck her head on a waterski.
    c. 46-year-old patient who had lacerations of the forehead in a motor-vehicle accident.
    d. 78-year-old patient who fell and hit his head on the floor but experienced only a slight headache.

54. A patient taking sertraline for depression noted a decrease in urinary output over a one-month period. The serum sodium level was 120 mEq/L (120 mmol/L). The patient exhibited mild confusion, anorexia, and nausea and was diagnosed with syndrome of inappropriate antidiuretic hormone secretion (SIADH). The sertraline, which is associated with hyponatremia, was discontinued and the patient's sodium levels are monitored. What first-line intervention should the AGACNP prescribe?

    a. Fluid limitation.
    b. IV sodium.
    c. Oral sodium.
    d. Loop diuretic.

55. A patient with end-stage renal disease develops a hypertensive crisis with the following vital signs: BP, 182/108; P, 104; R, 18; and oxygen saturation, 98%. The patient is anxious and complains of headache, but there is no indication of organ damage. The patient is administered labetalol by infusion. What percent reduction in BP should the patient have during the first 6 hours after treatment is initiated?

    a. 10%.
    b. 33%.
    c. 66%.
    d. 100%.

56. If a 64-year-old male African-American patient with diabetes has BP readings that average about 154/96, the first-line pharmacologic therapy that the AGACNP should advise is:

    a. thiazide diuretic or calcium channel blocker.
    b. angiotensin-converting enzyme (ACE) inhibitor and angiotensin II receptor blocker (ARB).
    c. thiazide diuretic or ARB.
    d. loop diuretic.

57. A 28-year-old female patient is recovering from a Zika infection and tells the AGACNP that she has been trying to conceive and that her male partner has been possibly exposed. Before trying to conceive again, the patient should be advised to wait at least:

    a. 4 weeks.
    b. 8 weeks.
    c. 6 months.
    d. 12 months.

58. If a Navajo patient tells the AGACNP that he has "ghost sickness," the most appropriate response is:

    a. "There is no such disease."
    b. "What do you mean?"
    c. "Is that a common name for a real illness?"
    d. "How does ghost sickness make you feel?"

59. A patient with hypertrophic cardiomyopathy has been prescribed propranolol. The AGACNP should inform the patient and family members that patients taking the drug are at risk for:

    a. tachycardia.
    b. depression.
    c. hypertension.
    d. anorexia.

60. A 68-year-old male in good health has a sudden onset of severe weakness, chest pain, dyspnea, cough, and low-grade fever of 38°C (100.4°F), The patient's systolic BP is palpable at 52 mm Hg; P, 128; R, 38; and oxygen saturation, 81% on room air. Which of the following tests may provide the best information to rule out pulmonary embolism?

    a. D-dimer assay.
    b. Arterial blood gases.
    c. Complete blood count (CBC).
    d. Partial thromboplastin time (PTT).

61. If a patient is diagnosed with tuberculosis and must take antituberculosis drugs, for which of the following should the AGACNP consider referral to the health department for directly observed therapy (DOT)?

    a. Patient has comorbidity with diabetes mellitus.
    b. Patient states he dislikes following any treatment regimen.
    c. Patient has a low income and lives in Section 8 housing.
    d. Patient is taking methadone for heroin addiction.

62. If the AGACNP notes that staffing patterns do not always match the workload in the acute care unit, the first step to a solution is to:

    a. complain to management.
    b. organize staff members to demand changes.
    c. determine how staffing decisions are made.
    d. prepare a list of potential changes.

63. A 56-year-old patient has symptoms consistent with cholecystitis. Which of the following is a differential diagnosis that should be considered?

    a. Cystitis.
    b. Acute gastritis.
    c. Liver carcinoma.
    d. Bowel obstruction.

64. According to the Payne-Martin classification system for skin tears, an example of a category II skin tear is which of the following?

    a. Scant tissue loss: Partial thickness injury and ≤25% of the epidermal flap lost.
    b. Linear: Full-thickness wound in a wrinkle or furrow with the epidermis and dermis pulled apart.
    c. Flap: Partial thickness wound with a flap that can cover a wound with ≤ 1 mm of dermis exposed.
    d. Complete partial-thickness injury with loss of the epidermal flap.

65. If the AGACNP observes an unlicensed assistive personnel (UAP) massaging the reddened heels of an immobile patient, the AGACNP should:

    a. file a complaint about the UAP's lack of competence.
    b. compliment the UAP for providing good preventive care.
    c. take no action because this is part of routine care.
    d. explain how massaging reddened tissue may cause tissue damage.

66. The hospital administration has collected patient surveys to determine the needs that patients feel are most important. The next step in the quality improvement process should be to:

    a. collect data regarding current status of these needs.
    b. determine measurable outcomes.
    c. develop a plan.
    d. assemble a multidisciplinary team.

67. If the AGACNP discovers that a patient faces various problems in returning home after discharge, including lack of adequate income and impaired ability to prepare food, and refers the patient to a social worker for assistance, the type of power that the AGACNP is exhibiting is:

    a. transformational power.
    b. advocacy power.
    c. affirmative power.
    d. integrative power.

68. When reviewing staffing needs, the AGACNP finds that staff members' time is most impacted by answering patients' call lights and responding to their needs. Which of the following strategies is likely to be most effective for time saving?

    a. Rounding on patients hourly.
    b. Grouping patients by severity.
    c. Reminding patients to use the call light only for medical needs.
    d. Assigning one staff member to answer call lights.

69. A patient who developed polyarthralgia was recently diagnosed with systemic lupus erythematosus. When educating the patient about lifestyle changes, the AGACNP should plan to include:

    a. dietary modifications.
    b. weight loss and exercise regimens.
    c. energy conservation and skin protection.
    d. bowel care regimens.

70. An 18-year-old football player experienced blunt trauma to his lower left leg during a tackle. The patient was able to walk initially with no difficulty. The patient comes to the hospital about an hour later, complaining of severe pain and tightness in the lower leg as well as a sensation of burning. The lower leg is edematous and the skin is taut, although a distal pulse is palpable and the capillary refill time is within normal limits. The priority intervention should be to:

    a. measure compartment pressure.
    b. order an X-ray of the leg.
    c. order a computerized tomography (CT) scan of the leg.
    d. apply ice packs and elevate the leg.

71. The AGACNP is caring for a patient with kidney failure. The patient's glomerular filtration rate (GFR) has been falling and is 28 ml/min/1.73^3. At what GFR should the AGACNP expect that the patient will need to begin renal replacement therapy?

    a. <30 mL/min/1.732.
    b. <25 mL/min/1.732.
    c. <20 mL/min/1.732.
    d. <15 mL/min/1.732.

72. A patient who experienced tonic-clonic seizures is newly diagnosed with epilepsy and has started on antiseizure medication. When the AGACNP is educating the patient about the disease, the most important advice is to:

    a. avoid all exercise.
    b. tell all family, friends, and associates about the diagnosis.
    c. follow a healthy lifestyle.
    d. never stop taking the medication abruptly.

73. Oxygen exchange in the lungs decreases with age because of:
   a. atrophy of the alveoli and alveolar ducts.
   b. enlargement of the alveoli and alveolar ducts.
   c. increased mucous production in the alveoli and alveolar ducts.
   d. decrease in the number of alveoli and alveolar ducts.

74. In evaluating research as part of the development of evidence-based practice guidelines, the four evaluative/trustworthiness criteria are (1) credibility, (2) dependability, (3) transferability, and (4):
   a. controllability.
   b. applicability.
   c. accountability.
   d. confirmability.

75. A 66-year-old male patient complains of increasing abdominal pain and has been passing 3 to 4 sticky, black, foul-smelling stools for 3 to 4 days. The patient's vital signs are BP, 116/78 supine; P, 112; R, 22; and temperature, 37°C (98.6°F). The standing BP dropped to 88/58, and the patient experienced dizziness. The patient's hemoglobin is 9.2 mg/dL (92 mmol/L), hematocrit is 28%, mean cell volume (MCV) is 70 fL, and BUN is 46 mg/dL (16.4 mmol/L). Based on these observations, the AGACNP should suspect:
   a. iron deficiency anemia and intestinal perforation.
   b. hemolytic anemia and gastritis.
   c. iron deficiency anemia and upper GI bleeding.
   d. iron deficiency anemia and lower GI bleeding.

76. A 30-year-old male patient is to be discharged after a vasectomy. When educating the patient, the AGACNP should stress the importance of:
   a. using an alternate form of contraception for 6 to 8 weeks.
   b. avoiding all sexual activity for up to 3 months.
   c. resuming normal sexual activity as soon as possible.
   d. anticipating erectile dysfunction for 6 to 8 weeks.

77. A patient recently returned from serving in the military in the Middle East is hospitalized with post-traumatic stress disorder (PTSD). The patient has recurring flashbacks and nightmares and is constantly vigilant and anxious. The patient tells the AGACNP repeatedly that he should have died with his friends. Which of the following is the most appropriate response?
   a. "You have a lot to live for."
   b. "You won't always feel that way, I'm sure."
   c. "Why do you feel that way?"
   d. "Are you thinking about killing yourself?"

78. The AGACNP is screening patients for referral to a case manager. Which of the following patients is most likely to benefit from case management?
   a. An 18-year-old patient with second-degree burns on the hands.
   b. A 62-year-old patient with repeated hospitalizations for chronic obstructive pulmonary disease (COPD) and diabetes.
   c. A 38-year-old patient after mastectomy for breast cancer.
   d. A 52-year-old patient after a knee replacement.

79. A patient with dilated cardiomyopathy is on the transplant list for a heart but none has become available. The patient's ejection fraction has fallen to 22%, and the patient's functional ability is markedly decreased. The AGACNP recognizes that the patient may benefit most from a(n):

    a. pacemaker.
    b. left ventricular assist device (LVAD).
    c. intra-aortic balloon pump (IABP).
    d. implantable cardioverter defibrillator (ICD).

80. A patient with chronic low back pain states that he wants to try complementary therapy to relieve pain because medications have been ineffective and asks the AGACNP which of the therapies are likely to relieve discomfort. The AGACNP should reply that the therapy that has documented effectiveness is:

    a. acupuncture.
    b. herbal medicines.
    c. homeopathic medicines.
    d. healing touch.

81. When the AGACNP is counseling a patient before surgery to remove a colon tumor and create a colostomy, the patient asks about whether stools will be regular after surgery. The AGACNP advises the patient that bowel regularity can be expected if the tumor is in:

    a. any part of the colon.
    b. the ascending or transverse colon.
    c. the transverse or descending colon.
    d. the descending colon or the rectum.

82. Which of the following terms refers specifically to the process by which a person is granted authority to practice in an organization?

    a. Licensing.
    b. Privileging.
    c. Credentialing.
    d. Certifying.

83. The primary criterion for referral to a hospice program is:

    a. Severe, intractable pain.
    b. Life-threatening disease.
    c. Probability that death will occur within 6 months.
    d. A do-not-resuscitate (DNR) order.

84. Which of the following legal procedures authorizes disclosure of patient personal health information?

    a. Subpoena.
    b. Subpoena duces tecum.
    c. Warrant.
    d. Court order.

85. Which of the following is an essential element when the AGACNP is using adult learning principles to work with adult learners?

    a. Collaboration.
    b. Direction.
    c. Assisted learning.
    d. Prompting.

86. The most effective method to ensure that team members in an acute care unit are prepared to carry out the disaster plan in case of an emergency is to:

    a. post guidelines in prominent spots.
    b. make the complete disaster plan readily available.
    c. schedule practice/simulation drills.
    d. remind staff to review disaster plans.

87. A patient with schizophrenia should be evaluated for which of the following common comorbidities?

    a. Conduct disorder.
    b. Depression.
    c. Eating disorder.
    d. Post-traumatic stress disorder (PTSD).

88. A nonverbal young adult patient with autism spectrum disorder is scheduled for a minor surgical procedure and is accompanied by a parent, but the patient is very frightened, distressed, and uncooperative. The best way to reduce the patient's anxiety is to:

    a. leave the patient alone for a period of time.
    b. pat the patient on the arm and speak soothingly.
    c. ask the parent for advice about appropriate interventions.
    d. ask the parent to leave the room.

89. A 59-year-old patient is admitted to the medical-surgical unit with pneumonia. Which of the following is a risk factor for the development of healthcare-associated pneumonia?

    a. Antibiotic therapy 120 days previously.
    b. History of an infected great toe 120 days previously.
    c. Home infusion therapy 70 to 75 days previously
    d. Acute hospitalization for 4 days 65 days previously.

90. When determining the level of risk for evaluation and management (E/M) services, which three components of the Centers for Medicare & Medicaid Services (CMS) Table of Risk must be considered?

    a. Presenting problem(s), diagnostic procedure(s) ordered, and management options selected.
    b. Social and personal history, physical exam, and medical necessity.
    c. Diagnosis, physical exam, and diagnostic procedure(s) ordered.
    d. Chief complaint, diagnostic procedure(s) ordered, and physical exam.

91. The coding system that is used to code for outpatient diagnoses is:

a. International Classification of Diseases, version 9 (ICD-9).
b. Healthcare Common Procedure Coding System (HCPCS)/American Medical Association's Current Procedural Terminology (CPT).
c. ICD-10-CM.
d. ICD-10-PCS.

92. A patient brought to the emergency department after a motorcycle accident exhibits bruising over the area of the mastoid process (Battle's sign) and well as otorrhea. These are indications of:

a. cervical injury.
b. basilar skull fracture.
c. epidural hematoma.
d. subarachnoid hemorrhage.

93. Risk factors commonly associated with development of diabetes mellitus, type 2, include:

a. young age and inactivity.
b. malnutrition and anemia.
c. obesity and inactivity.
d. smoking and drinking alcohol.

94. A male patient is considered at high risk for health problems if his waist-to-hip ratio is greater than:

a. 0.8.
b. 0.9.
c. 0.95.
d. 1.0.

95. Which of the following types of fractures is likely to result in the greatest loss of blood?

a. femur.
b. pelvis.
c. elbow.
d. tibia.

96. If an older patient complains of urinary frequency and urgency, increasing shortness of breath, pain in the right knee when walking prolonged distances, and chronic constipation, the order of priority (most critical to least) should be:

a. (1) urinary frequency and urgency, (2) shortness of breath, (3) pain in the right knee, and (4) chronic constipation.
b. (1) chronic constipation, (2) shortness of breath, (3) urinary frequency and urgency, and (4) pain in the right knee.
c. (1) shortness of breath, (2) urinary frequency and urgency, (3) chronic constipation, and (4) pain in the right knee.
d. (1) pain in right knee, (2) shortness of breath, (3) urinary frequency and urgency, and (4) chronic constipation.

97. If an AGACNP copies and pastes free text from one patient's electronic health record (EHR) to another when the information needed is similar, this procedure:

a. is a dangerous practice.
b. is a good time-saving method.
c. should be first authorized by the medical staff.
d. helps standardize documentation.

98. Although shared governance focuses primarily on empowering nursing, partnership councils focus on:

a. physicians.
b. nonmedical personnel.
c. members at all levels.
d. department heads.

99. A 72-year-old patient complains of increasing fatigue, weakness, and dyspnea on exertion and lack of interest in activities. The patient's pulse rate shows increases from 70 to 96, blood pressure from 126/78 to 150/96 and respirations from 18 to 26 three minutes after activity; a likely nursing diagnosis is:

a. risk-prone health behaviors.
b. ineffective coping.
c. activity intolerance.
d. anxiety.

100. Patients who are taking phenytoin for seizure disorders should be advised to have regular dental care because of an increased risk of:

a. caries.
b. gingival hyperplasia.
c. tooth staining.
d. abscesses.

101. When assessing for facial palsy as part of the National Institutes of Health (NIH) Stroke Scale, which part of the face is the best place to focus on for minor paralysis?

a. Mouth.
b. Forehead.
c. Eyebrows.
d. Eyes.

102. When the AGACNP is screening telephone calls in the acute care telehealth program, a patient calls to complain of low back pain. Which of the following additional symptoms represents an emergent situation and should result in the AGACNP advising the patient to hang up and call 9-1-1?

a. Pain radiating down the left leg.
b. Fever of 38°C/100.4°F.
c. Sudden loss of bowel and bladder control.
d. Burning on urination and frequency.

103. An example of tertiary prevention for patients with diabetes mellitus is:

    a. achieving A1c target.
    b. yearly flu vaccine.
    c. annual screening for kidney disease.
    d. low-sodium diet.

104. Which of the following is a differential diagnosis that must be ruled out for a patient presenting with possible stroke because of a sudden onset of decreased level of consciousness and unilateral weakness?

    a. hyperglycemia.
    b. hypoglycemia.
    c. Lyme disease.
    d. Guillain-Barré syndrome.

105. The primary purpose of conducting a problem-based assessment of a patient is to:

    a. focus on one problem.
    b. review one body system.
    c. focus on the patient history.
    d. create a problem list.

106. In a patient with onset of myasthenia gravis at age 38, which organ probably triggered the autoimmune response?

    a. Thymus.
    b. Spleen.
    c. Pituitary gland.
    d. Thyroid gland.

107. The AGACNP is concerned that an older patient who fractured a femur in a fall may be drinking excessively. Which of the following tools may be most appropriate for assessment?

    a. Healthy Living Questionnaire.
    b. Geriatric Depression Scale (GDS).
    c. Quality of Life Scale.
    d. CAGE Assessment.

108. If, when using the Plan-Do-Study-Act (PDSA) method of continuous quality improvement, study of the outcomes of a trial indicates that the solution that was instituted was not effective, the next step is to:

    a. return to the plan step.
    b. return to the do step.
    c. discontinue the process.
    d. continue to the act step.

109. The end diastolic volume of the heart minus the end-systolic volume equals the:

    a. cardiac output.
    b. stroke volume.
    c. preload.
    d. afterload.

110. A 42-year-old male comes to the emergency department with slight jaundice and complaining of clay-colored stools and flu-like symptoms. The primary tests that screen for hepatitis include:

a. alanine transaminase (ALT) and aspartate transaminase (AST).
b. complete blood count (CBC) and differential.
c. bilirubin and lactate dehydrogenase (LDH).
d. total protein and serum ammonia.

111. When counseling a 26-year-old patient with condylomata acuminata (genital warts), the AGACNP notes that the treatment with the highest success rate is:

a. podophyllin/Podofilox.
b. infrared coagulation.
c. surgical excision.
d. cryosurgery.

112. Lipid screening should be done every 5 years starting at age:

a. 60.
b. 45.
c. 30.
d. 20.

113. When performing medication reconciliation for a geriatric patient, the AGACNP is concerned that some medications or dosages may be inappropriate for older patients. The most efficient method of checking these medications is probably to consult:

a. the Physicians' Desk Reference (PDR).
b. Drugs.com.
c. the Beers Criteria.
d. drug manufacturers.

114. Which of the following puts a 17-year-old patient at risk for oral cancer?

a. Chewing sugar-free gum.
b. Smoking electronic cigarettes.
c. Drinking carbonated beverages.
d. Drinking caffeinated beverages.

115. A 36-year-old HIV-positive patient is being tested for tuberculosis (TB) with a tuberculin skin test. A positive reaction for an HIV patient is induration of:

a. ≥5 mm.
b. ≥8 mm.
c. ≥10 mm.
d. ≥15 mm.

116. If an older female patient with moderately advanced dementia is cradling a doll and says, "This is my baby," and refuses to relinquish the doll for an examination, the most appropriate response is:

a. "That is a doll and not a baby."
b. "I'll hold the baby for you."
c. "I won't bother your baby."
d. "You must give me the doll."

117. Which of the following heart sounds is an indication of heart failure in an older adult?

    a. Opening snap.
    b. Ejection click.
    c. Friction rub.
    d. S3.

118. Which of the following treatments commonly prescribed for fibromyalgia is believed to decrease pain by reducing electrical activity associated with overactive nerve impulses?

    a. Duloxetine (Cymbalta).
    b. Pregabalin (Lyrica).
    c. Milnacipran HCL (Savella).
    d. Gabapentin (Neurontin).

119. A 42-year-old patient with chronic lymphocytic leukemia (CLL) has developed thrombocytopenia. At what platelet count would the patient likely begin to exhibit petechiae, nasal bleeding, and gingival bleeding?

    a. 100,000.
    b. 50,000.
    c. 18,000.
    d. 5,000.

120. A palliative care patient has been drinking heavily and smoking. He states that he has been having severe episodes of chest pain about the same time each afternoon when he is watching television. Which diagnosis is most likely?

    a. Esophageal varices.
    b. Stable angina.
    c. Unstable angina.
    d. Variant (Prinzmetal's) angina.

121. Which of the following should require input from all members of the interdisciplinary team (IDT)?

    a. Titrating pain medications.
    b. Developing the plan of care.
    c. Instructing the patient in stress reduction techniques.
    d. Managing skin care.

122. According to the modified Wagner foot ulcer classification system, a full-thickness ulcer that extends to the tendon or joint but without abscess or osteomyelitis is classified as:

    a. grade 1.
    b. grade 2.
    c. grade 3.
    d. grade 4.

123. An older adult with a urinary infection may exhibit:

    a. confusion.
    b. hallucinations.
    c. depression.
    d. anxiety.

124. Which of the following statements by an AGACNP demonstrates a good understanding of peer review?

    a. "I don't mind reviewing someone as long as my review is anonymous."
    b. "My peer review is going to get him fired for incompetence!"
    c. "Peer review is a good learning experience for me and the person I'm reviewing."
    d. "The supervisor should do the peer reviews because the supervisor has more authority."

125. A 34-year-old male patient who returned from military service in Afghanistan has begun to have severe, frightening flashbacks related to post-traumatic stress disorder (PTSD). If the AGACNP finds the patient cowering in the corner of the room in a state of panic, the best approach is to say:

    a. "Give me your hand and I'll help you up."
    b. "I know you are afraid, but you are safe here."
    c. "Just deep-breathe and relax."
    d. "There is nothing to be afraid of."

126. If an insurer, such as Blue Cross/Blue Shield, denies a claim, within how many days of denial must an internal appeal be submitted?

    a. 30.
    b. 60.
    c. 90.
    d. 180.

127. Which of the following tests used to assess cognitive abilities for a patient with dementia includes remembering and later repeating the names of three common objects and drawing the face of a clock with all 12 numbers and the two hands indicating a specified time?

    a. Mini-Mental State Examination (MMSE).
    b. Mini-Cog.
    c. Instrumental Activities of Daily Living (IADLs) scale.
    d. Confusion Assessment Method.

128. A 70-year-old male in good health except for high blood pressure reported a sudden weakness and loss of movement and sensation in his right arm and leg, persisting for about 5 minutes. A carotid bruit is found on examination, but he has had no further symptoms. Which type of assessment to confirm transient ischemic attack is most indicated initially?

    a. Magnetic resonance imaging (MRI) of the neck and brain.
    b. Noncontrast computed tomography (CT) of the brain.
    c. Carotid angiography, including digital subtraction angiography.
    d. Transesophageal echocardiography.

129. Which of the following presents a barrier to systems thinking?

    a. Reliance on past experience.
    b. Identification with purpose.
    c. Strong consensus.
    d. Adaptability.

130. In developing evidence-based guidelines to reduce urinary tract infections in patients with indwelling catheters, which of the following should carry the most weight in developing new policies?

    a. Best practices identified through literature review.
    b. Nursing staff preferences.
    c. Physician preference.
    d. Cost-effectiveness.

131. A 38-year-old female patient has had recurrent struvite (magnesium ammonium phosphate) urinary stones. The most appropriate treatment regimen includes:

    a. increased hydration and thiazide diuretic.
    b. antibiotics and acetohydroxamic acid.
    c. increased hydration and potassium citrate.
    d. alpha-penicillamine and tiopronin.

132. The most important factor in cost management is:

    a. purchasing in bulk and limiting choices in equipment and supplies.
    b. conducting cost comparisons and choosing the least expensive options.
    c. providing the minimal care necessary to achieve acceptable outcomes.
    d. eliminating duplication of services and care fragmentation.

133. Which of the following is an example of documentation that is currently on The Joint Commission's "Do Not Use" list?

    a. 5 mg.
    b. 0.5 mg.
    c. 15 U.
    d. @.

134. A 50-year-old female complains of recent bouts of palpitations, restlessness, and anxiety. Her skin is dry, and she complains of an inability to tolerate excess heat or cold, difficulty sleeping, and constipation. Thyroid function tests indicate a decrease in thyroid-stimulating hormone (TSH) but increases in both triiodothyronine (T3) and its prohormone, thyroxine (T4). Which medication should the AGACNP prescribe for the patient to take while arranging for a referral to an endocrinologist?

    a. Levothyroxine (Synthroid).
    b. Metoprolol (Lopressor).
    c. Methimazole (Tapazole).
    d. Propylthiouracil.

135. A patient has chest pain, dyspnea, and hypotension. A 12-lead electrocardiogram (ECG) shows atrial rates of 250 with regular ventricular rates of 100. P waves are saw-toothed (referred to as F waves), QRS shape and duration (0.4 to 0.11 seconds) are normal, the PR interval is hard to calculate because of F waves, and the P:QRS ratio is 2–4:1. Which of the following diagnoses fits this profile?

    a. Premature atrial contraction.
    b. Premature junctional contraction.
    c. Atrial fibrillation.
    d. Atrial flutter.

136. Which of the following is a common nondisease cause of illness?

    a. Immobility.
    b. Worry.
    c. Vegan diet.
    d. Jogging.

137. A homeless patient complains of severe pruritis about the wrists, between the fingers, on the elbows, and about the penis and scrotum, worsening at night, with the areas reddened and excoriated from scratching. The most likely diagnosis is:

    a. scabies.
    b. tinea cruris.
    c. pediculosis corporis.
    d. psoriasis.

138. Which of the following is the correct procedure to evaluate the function of cranial nerve X (vagus)?

    a. Ask the patient to protrude the tongue and move it from side to side against a tongue depressor.
    b. Observe patient swallowing, and place sugar or salt at the back third of the tongue to determine if the patient can differentiate.
    c. Ask the patient to swallow and speak, and place a tongue blade on the posterior tongue or pharynx to elicit the gag reflex.
    d. Place hands on patient's shoulders and ask the patient to shrug against resistance.

139. Which of the following bacterial infections is most often associated with the development of Guillain-Barré syndrome?

    a. Salmonella.
    b. Shigella.
    c. Mycoplasma pneumoniae.
    d. Campylobacter jejuni.

140. Because there is only one bed available but two patients in need of care, the AGACNP recommends that one patient be transferred to another facility. The decision regarding which patient to transfer should be based on which ethical principle?

    a. Nonmaleficence.
    b. Beneficence.
    c. Justice.
    d. Autonomy.

141. For Medicare reimbursement, if a physician received $200 for a procedure (out of a $240 charge), what percentage of the amount the physician received would the AGACNP receive when billing Medicare for the same procedure?

    a. 75%.
    b. 80%.
    c. 85%.
    d. 90%.

142. A patient with a history of alcoholism and cirrhosis has signs of portal hypertension, including abdominal ascites. The patient should be assessed for:

a. thrombocytosis.
b. esophageal/gastric varices.
c. seizure disorder.
d. muscle hypertrophy.

143. The AGACNP should recommend the pneumococcal conjugate vaccination (PCV13) to:

a. all adolescents and adults.
b. adults age 30 and older.
c. adults age 60 and older.
d. adults age 65 and older.

144. Because of high risk, the AGACNP should screen bariatric patients for:

a. depression and eating disorders.
b. bipolar disorder and schizophrenia.
c. domestic partner abuse.
d. neurological disorders.

145. A trauma patient has lost 15% to 25% (750–1500 mL) of total blood volume and exhibits tachycardia (110 bpm), prolonged capillary refill, and increased diastolic BP. Respirations are 24, and urinary output is 25 mL/hr. This hemorrhagic shock is classified as:

a. class I.
b. class II.
c. class III.
d. class IV.

146. A patient is hospitalized with an acute myocardial infarction with ST segment elevation. A 50% reduction in mortality rates occurs if the patient is treated with thrombolytic therapy within:

a. 12 hours.
b. 6 hours.
c. 3 hours.
d. 10 minutes.

147. A patient presents in the emergency department after falling from a horse and being kicked in the left side. In addition to a fractured left lower rib, the patient exhibits elevation of the left hemidiaphragm, left lower lobe atelectasis, and pleural effusion as well as tachycardia, hypotension, left flank pain, and positive Kehr's sign (pain referred to the left shoulder). The AGACNP recognizes these signs and symptoms as being indications of:

a. ruptured spleen.
b. hepatic trauma.
c. gastric perforation.
d. pancreatic trauma.

148. Respiratory alkalosis almost always results from:

a. base bicarbonate deficit.
b. base bicarbonate excess.
c. hypoventilation.
d. hyperventilation.

149. Which of the following precipitating factors for angina results in release of catecholamines (which increase the heart rate and cause vasoconstriction) as well as a decrease in available oxygen to the heart because of increased carbon monoxide levels?

    a. Nicotine (smoking).
    b. Exertion.
    c. Temperature extremes.
    d. Sexual activity.

150. An exercise electrocardiogram (ECG) (stress test) is contraindicated for a patient who:

    a. has taken sildenafil citrate (Viagra) a day previously.
    b. has chest pain at rest or on minimal exertion.
    c. has a history of cardiac dysrhythmias.
    d. receives antihypertensive drugs.

151. A male patient with a history of antisocial personality disorder asks the female AGACNP if she spent the weekend with her boyfriend. The most appropriate response is:

    a. "I don't discuss my dates with patients."
    b. "It's not appropriate to ask the nursing staff personal questions."
    c. "You're going to have to stay in your room if you continue asking personal questions."
    d. "That's none of your business!"

152. Which of the following drugs is generally most effective for treatment of trigeminal neuralgia?

    a. Baclofen.
    b. Phenytoin.
    c. Gabapentin.
    d. Carbamazepine.

153. The AGACNP may consider ordering a magnetic resonance imaging (MRI) scan to screen for breast cancer for:

    a. all women.
    b. women older than 55.
    c. women with >20% lifetime risk of breast cancer.
    d. with >15% risk of breast cancer.

154. A 27-year-old male with lower back pain and stiffness that improve with activity but are progressing upward is diagnosed with ankylosing spondylitis. The initial treatment regimen includes:

    a. NSAIDs.
    b. Tumor necrosis factor (TNF) inhibitors.
    c. corticosteroids.
    d. statins.

155. The most common cause of medical error is:

    a. lack of knowledge.
    b. inadequate procedures.
    c. staffing patterns.
    d. communication problems.

156. Which of the following antibiotics is the drug of choice for mild to moderate *Clostridium difficile* infection?

    a. Ampicillin.
    b. Metronidazole.
    c. Erythromycin.
    d. Vancomycin.

157. When the AGACNP is educating a patient with a familial history of rheumatoid arthritis (RA), the patient should be advised to:

    a. stop smoking.
    b. stop drinking alcohol.
    c. limit exercise.
    d. avoid drinking tea.

158. If a patient has complaints of postoperative pain, which of the following is an example of a cause-focused action as opposed to a solution-focused action?

    a. Administer pain medication to the patient.
    b. Instruct the patient in visualization and relaxation.
    c. Examine the wound for signs of infection or complications.
    d. Order a stronger pain medication.

159. In response to decreased renal perfusion or decreased sodium intake, the kidneys secrete:

    a. aldosterone.
    b. angiotensinogen.
    c. angiotensin I.
    d. renin.

160. If a coworker claims to have disposed of narcotics without a witness and asks the AGACNP to sign after the fact, the most appropriate action is to:

    a. sign if the person is known and trusted.
    b. refuse to sign because it would constitute complicity.
    c. consider the circumstances before deciding.
    d. notify the Drug Enforcement Agency (DEA) of a violation.

161. A patient is airlifted to the hospital with a spinal cord injury and is not breathing independently. Total loss of respiratory muscle function occurs with spinal cord injuries above:

    a. C4.
    b. C5.
    c. C6.
    d. C7

162. Which of the following lifestyle changes should the AGACNP recommend to a patient with obstructive sleep apnea?

    a. Stop all use of alcohol.
    b. Move to a different climate.
    c. Stop smoking.
    d. Sleep only sitting in a chair.

163. A 40-year-old patient is diagnosed with latent autoimmune diabetes in adults (LADA) (aka as "slow diabetes" or "diabetes 1.5"). The duration of time from onset of symptoms to insulin dependence is usually about:

    a. 6 months.
    b. 18 months.
    c. 24 months.
    d. 2 to 4 years.

164. Which of the following types of dressings is most effective for infected wounds with large amounts of drainage?

    a. Hydrocolloid.
    b. Alginate.
    c. Hydrogel.
    d. Polyamide net.

165. A patient has acute pancreatitis and has an order for a histamine-2 receptor antagonist (ranitidine). The purpose of prescribing this drug is to:

    a. decrease hydrochloric acid (HCL) secretion.
    b. relieve pain.
    c. decrease vagal stimulation.
    d. relax smooth muscles.

166. A 16-year-old patient experienced a concussion when he was tackled by another player while playing football. The patient lost consciousness for about 20 seconds and has some persistent confusion after 30 minutes. The concussion would be classified as:

    a. ungraded.
    b. grade 1.
    c. grade 2.
    d. grade 3.

167. During which phase of the healing process does the AGACNP expect a wound to begin to form granulation tissue?

    a. Phase I: Hemostasis.
    b. Phase II: Inflammation.
    c. Phase III: Proliferation.
    d. Phase IV: Maturation.

168. Which class of compression stocking is appropriate for prevention of venous ulcers in patients at risk?

    a. Class I: 20 to 30 mm Hg.
    b. Class 2: 30 to 40 mm Hg.
    c. Class 3: 40 to 50 mm Hg.
    d. Class 4: 50 to 60 mm Hg.

169. A 33-year-old patient developed hemorrhagic colitis after ingesting *Escherichia coli* (Shiga toxin-producing *E. coli* [STEC] O157:H7) in contaminated produce during a recent outbreak. Which of the following treatments is indicated?

    a. Supportive care only.
    b. IV antibiotics.
    c. Immunoglobulin.
    d. Corticosteroids.

170. A patient is admitted with possible Guillain-Barré syndrome (GBS) because of respiratory distress and weakness. The AGACNP recognizes that the weakness that is characteristic of GBS is:

    a. descending and symmetrical.
    b. descending and asymmetrical.
    c. ascending and asymmetrical.
    d. ascending and symmetrical.

171. A patient reports the sudden appearance of a large number of cherry angiomas on her abdomen. The AGACNP recognizes that this may be a sign of:

    a. sun exposure.
    b. circulatory impairment.
    c. internal malignancy.
    d. internal infection.

172. A 72-year-old stroke patient has daily physical therapy that includes assisted walking on a treadmill. A large mirror is placed in front of the treadmill. The purpose of the mirror is to:

    a. provide visual feedback.
    b. distract the patient during exercise.
    c. reassure the patient that he won't fall.
    d. prevent claustrophobia.

173. If the AGACNP prescribes disulfiram to a patient for alcohol dependence, the patient should be advised that, after stopping the medication, a disulfiram-alcohol reaction can occur for up to:

    a. 24 to 48 hours.
    b. 3 to 4 days.
    c. 1 week.
    d. 2 weeks.

174. A patient with obsessive-compulsive disorder is hospitalized with a myocardial infarction (MI) and uses ritualized number patterns of behavior, such as emptying water out of a glass four times before drinking from the glass. The AGACNP recognizes that the primary rationale for this behavior is to:

    a. annoy staff members.
    b. reduce anxiety.
    c. respond to delusions.
    d. maintain control.

175. When treating a patient for increased intracranial pressure (ICP), the goal should be to maintain the ICP within normal range and the cerebral perfusion pressure (CPP) at:

    a. >40 mm Hg.
    b. >50 mm Hg.
    c. >60 mm Hg.
    d. >80 mm Hg.

176. When describing chest pain, the patient runs the fingers of both hands up and down either side of the sternum. The most likely origin of the pain is:

    a. gastrointestinal (GI) system.
    b. cardiovascular ischemia.
    c. pulmonary embolism.
    d. aortic dissection.

177. When educating a patient with coronary artery disease about managing anginal episodes, the AGACNP advises the patient to:

    a. take nitroglycerin three times 5 minutes apart before calling 9-1-1 if pain persists.
    b. take nitroglycerin two times 5 minutes apart before calling 9-1-1 prior to the third dose if pain persists.
    c. take nitroglycerin one time and then call 9-1-1 prior to the second dose if the pain persists.
    d. call 9-1-1 before taking any doses of nitroglycerin.

178. Which of the following risk factors places a female patient at highest risk for a cardiovascular disease?

    a. Smoking.
    b. Diabetes mellitus.
    c. Obesity.
    d. Hypertension.

179. A patient involved in a frontal impact motor vehicle accident arrives at the emergency department with a markedly widened mediastinum, left hemothorax, and transient hypotension. Based on these findings, the AGACNP alerts staff that the patient likely has:

    a. cardiac tamponade.
    b. pulmonary embolism.
    c. flail chest.
    d. aortic rupture.

180. A certified nursing assistant (CNA) tells the AGACNP that when doing range-of-motion (ROM) exercises on a bedridden patient, the CNA meets resistance when trying to completely extend the right elbow. The AGACNP should advise the CNA to:

    a. avoid doing ROM exercises on the right arm.
    b. force the arm into complete extension.
    c. extend the arm slightly beyond the point of resistance.
    d. extend the arm only to the point of resistance.

181. When discussing safety issues with team members, the AGACNP reminds the team that the best way to prevent falls is to:

    a. use strategies appropriate for each patient.
    b. use restraints and side rails.
    c. keep the environment clean and neat.
    d. use a consistent approach for all patients.

182. If a patient hospitalized with an ischemic stroke develops a hypertensive emergency, the recommended drug treatment includes:

    a. nitroprusside.
    b. nicardipine.
    c. methyldopa.
    d. nitroglycerin.

183. In an emergency/disaster situation in which there are numerous casualties, which color code is used to indicate minor injuries (such as sprains and contusions) that can wait for medical care?

    a. Black.
    b. Yellow.
    c. Red.
    d. Green.

184. A 42-year-old male patient accidentally severed his right thumb above the knuckle, but surgeons were able to surgically reattach the digit. However, because the arteries but not the veins were reattached, the thumb became congested with blood, and leech therapy was instituted every 2 hours for 15- to 20-minute treatments. Following leech application, the patient should be observed:

    a. continuously.
    b. every 5 minutes.
    c. at the midpoint of treatment.
    d. at the end of treatment.

185. During a patient's physical examination, the AGACNP asks the patient to frown, smile, close eyes tightly against resistance, show teeth, lift eyebrows, and puff out the cheeks and hold against resistance. The cranial nerve that the AGACNP is assessing is:

    a. cranial nerve V.
    b. cranial nerve VI.
    c. cranial nerve VII.
    d. cranial nerve VIII.

186. With chronic mitral regurgitation, the heart chamber that enlarges first is the:

    a. right atrium.
    b. left atrium.
    c. right ventricle.
    d. left ventricle.

187. A 64-year-old male patient with cirrhosis of the liver has developed gynecomastia. The primary reason is:

    a. increased production of estrogen.
    b. edema in the breast tissue.
    c. impaired ability to metabolize estrogen.
    d. inflammation in the breast tissue.

188. A patient who has had a pacemaker implanted for bradycardia is to be discharged and asks the AGACNP about driving. The patient should be advised to avoid driving for:

    a. 24 to 48 hours.
    b. 1 week.
    c. 2 weeks.
    d. 1 month.

189. An abdominal CT has indicated that a patient has a large tumor low in the descending colon. The signs and symptoms that are characteristic of a tumor in this area include:

    a. pain, change in bowel habits, and bright-red blood in the stool.
    b. pain, distension, foul-smelling stool.
    c. pain; change in bowel habits; and black, tarry stool.
    d. pain, constipation, and fecal incontinence.

190. When initiating digoxin therapy for heart failure, the blood level of the drug should be measured within:

    a. 24 hours.
    b. 2 to 3 days.
    c. 1 to 2 weeks.
    d. 1 month.

191. A 17-year-old male patient who is tall with abnormally long arms, legs, and fingers and also has a chest abnormality (pectus excavatum) is diagnosed with Marfan syndrome. Which routine annual surveillance is indicated?

    a. Echocardiogram and complete metabolic panel.
    b. Eye exam and echocardiogram.
    c. Eye, orthopedic, and dental exams.
    d. Echocardiogram and dental exam.

192. A 58-year-old patient was admitted with severe acute pancreatitis. Which of the following findings 24 hours after admission and beginning of treatment indicates a worsening prognosis?

    a. Hematocrit drop of greater than 10%.
    b. Increase in blood urea nitrogen (BUN) greater than 2 g/dL.
    c. Serum calcium less than 10 mg/dL.
    d. Arterial PO2 of less than 65 mg/dL.

193. A 26-year-old patient has symptoms of chronic endometriosis with pelvic pain, dysmenorrhea, and dyspareunia. The imaging modality of choice for diagnosis is:

    a. X-ray.
    b. computed tomography (CT).
    c. magnetic resonance imaging (MRI).
    d. transvaginal ultrasonography.

194. A recent outbreak of giardiasis infection from an infected public pool has brought many patients to the emergency department. The public should be advised that, after ingestion of cysts, symptoms usually begin within:

    a. 24 to 48 hours.
    b. 1 to 2 days.
    c. 1 to 2 weeks.
    d. 3 to 4 weeks.

195. When conducting a physical examination of a 50-year-old patient, the AGACNP notes that the patient has spoon-shaped nails. This most commonly indicates:

    a. psoriasis.
    b. iron deficiency anemia.
    c. hypoxia.
    d. traumatic injury.

196. A patient with cervical cancer is treated with high-dose radiation (HDR) brachytherapy (intracavity). What other interventions are necessary during the 72 hours of treatment?

    a. Bedrest, low-residue diet, antidiarrheal medication, and indwelling urinary catheter.
    b. Bedrest, normal diet, stool softener, and bedpan privileges.
    c. Liquid diet and bathroom privileges.
    d. Bedrest, stool softener, liquid diet, and indwelling catheter.

197. If a patient has a scattered red rash with lesions that are less than 1 cm, flat, and nonpalpable with a circumscribed border, the rash would be described as:

    a. vesicular.
    b. nodular.
    c. papular.
    d. macular.

198. If a patient's nursing diagnosis is "Ineffective airway clearance associated with edema and effects of smoke inhalation," the goal should be to:

    a. Restore perfusion to lungs and vital organs.
    b. Reduce the risk of respiratory complications.
    c. Maintain a patent airway and adequate airway clearance.
    d. Achieve rapid reduction of airway edema.

199. Which of the following is the most common cause of visual loss for people over age 60 in the United States?

    a. Cataracts.
    b. Macular degeneration.
    c. Glaucoma.
    d. Retinal detachment.

200. A female carrier of the FMR1 gene for fragile X disorder is diagnosed with fragile X-associated primary ovarian insufficiency. This condition is characterized by:

    a. subfertility, infertility, and late-onset menopause.
    b. infertility and no onset of menses.
    c. subfertility, infertility, and early-onset menopause.
    d. subfertility and serial miscarriages.

Answers and Explanations

1. B: Patients with severe nausea and vomiting not associated with pain are most at risk for hypokalemia as well as azotemia and metabolic alkalosis. When the nausea and vomiting occur without pain, then the cause may be food poisoning, drugs, or gastroenteritis. Patients may become severely dehydrated. The normal potassium (K) value is 3.5 to 5.5 mEq/L. Hypoglycemia is <3.5 mEq/L with <2.5 mEq/L being the critical value. Signs and symptoms of hypokalemia include lethargy, weakness, nausea, vomiting, paresthesias, dysrhythmias, muscle cramps, hyporeflexia, hypotension, and tetany.

2. C: If a 54-year-old patient is to begin a short-term sleeping aid, such as eszopiclone (Lunesta), the AGACNP should document warning the patient to avoid operating heavy machinery or driving. Patients may have some residual daytime grogginess that can impair functioning and increase the risk of injury to self or others. Older adults may require a lesser dosage and may have increased drowsiness. Multiple drug interactions may occur with sleeping aids and other drugs.

3. D: Protamine sulfate, a heparin antagonist, is composed of strongly basic proteins derived from salmon sperm and some other fish, so allergies to fish can put the patient at risk for protamine anaphylactic reaction. Symptoms include the following:

- Sudden onset of weakness, dizziness, confusion.
- Urticaria
- Increased permeability of vascular system and loss of vascular tone.
- Severe hypotension leading to shock.
- Laryngospasm/bronchospasm with obstruction of airway causing dyspnea and wheezing.
- Nausea, vomiting, and diarrhea.
- Seizures, coma, and death.

4. A: Pharmacokinetics refers to the effects the body has on a drug, relating to the administration route, absorption dosage, administration frequency, mode of distribution, and serum levels. Pharmacokinetics must include consideration of the rate of clearance of the drug from the body and the mechanism of clearance (most commonly through the kidneys) as well as the dosage required to provide therapeutic benefits. Pharmacodynamics refers to the effects the drug has on the body.

5. B: Because the patient's sexual history shows risk for STDs, the patient's symptoms (purulent urethral discharge and urinary frequency and burning) are consistent with uncomplicated gonorrhea, and *Neisseria gonorrhoeae* is a Gram-negative diplococcus (consistent with Gram stain findings), the Centers for Disease Control and Prevention (CDC) recommends immediate treatment. Current drugs of choice for uncomplicated gonorrhea include cefatrizine (IM) and azithromycin (po), both in single doses. The culture and sensitivity results should be reviewed when available because of the risk of drug-resistant strains.

6. D: Pulsus paradoxus is a systolic blood pressure markedly lower during inhalation than exhalation. Pulsus paradoxus with >10 mm Hg difference is considered abnormal and is a common sign of cardiac tamponade. A decrease in blood pressure ≤10 mm Hg during inspiration is a normal finding, but increased pressure difference may indicate a number of cardiopulmonary complications, including pericardial effusion, pericarditis, pulmonary embolism, cardiogenic shock, chronic obstructive pulmonary disease (COPD), asthma, and obstruction of the superior vena cava. Blood pressure should be reevaluated if pulsus paradoxus is found to ensure correct readings.

- 33 -

7. C: RIFLE classifications (in order) include risk, injury, failure, loss, and end-stage kidney disease (ESKD). Injury includes increased serum creatinine by 200% or decreased glomerular filtration rate by >50% with urine output of <0.5 mL/kg/hr. over 12 hours. Risk (most common) includes increased serum creatinine by 150% or decreased GFR by >25% with urinary output of <0.5 mL/kg/r over 6 hours. Failure includes increased serum creatinine by 300% or decreased GFR by >75 or serum creatinine >4 mg/dL or an acute rise in serum creatinine >0.5 mg/dL with urine output <0.3 mL/kg/hr over 24 hours. Loss is acute renal failure persisting >4 weeks and ESKD >3 months.

8. A: AIDS is an example of a dementia-associated condition result from an environmental cause. Other examples include alcohol abuse, syphilis, vitamin deficiencies, and variant Creutzfeldt-Jakob disease. Other causes of dementia include organic (Alzheimer's disease, Parkinson's disease, normal pressure hydrocephalus), genetic (Huntington's disease), and traumatic (repeated head injuries, traumatic brain injuries). Alzheimer's disease is the most common cause of dementia in the elderly, accounting for 60% to 80% of cases of dementia in this population.

9. B: If, on assessment, the AGACNP observes that an 82-year-old patient has bruises on both forearms and her face, and the patient admits that her daughter sometimes gets angry and hits her but "feels terrible afterward," the AGACNP, as a mandatory reporter of child and elder abuse, should report the abuse to the appropriate authorities, even if the patient asks that the AGACNP not do so.

10. D: The critical value of serum pH is <7.20, the point at which adverse effects occur. Patients who are heavily sedated and not compensating with respirations may develop decreased sodium bicarbonate and acidic pH. Metabolic acidosis may result in decreased contractility and cardiac output with a subsequent reduction in blood flow to the liver and kidneys, increased pulmonary vascular resistance (PVR), vasoconstriction and arteriolar dilation, increased arrhythmias and ventricular fibrillation, dyspnea, tachypnea, hyperglycemia, hyperkalemia, increased production of lactate, and increased metabolic demands.

11. C: A good strategy for helping a client overcome feelings of low self-esteem includes providing opportunities for the client to make decisions. Other strategies include providing companionship and listening and encouraging the client to express her feelings and concerns. Positive feedback and praise should be given when earned rather than praising everything. Telling the client she has no reason to be depressed will invalidate her feelings and further lower her self-esteem. Low self-esteem is common among older adults because they have to deal with so many losses. They may become depressed, passive, and dependent.

12. B: If a 70-year-old male patient is admitted with right-sided heart failure, findings that are consistent with this diagnosis include increased jugular venous pressure. Hepatomegaly is also common with right-sided failure because the right side of the heart can't effectively receive and pump venous blood. Fluid retention, especially in the abdomen and lower extremities, may occur. Right-sided failure often follows left-sided failure, so patients have symptoms consistent with both right and left failure. Left-sided failure is most characterized by dyspnea because of low cardiac output and increased pulmonary venous congestion.

13. A: "The law doesn't allow me to give out any information about patients in order to protect their privacy and safety" is accurate and appropriate. The Health Insurance Portability and Accountability Act (HIPAA) addresses the privacy of health information. The AGACNP must not release any information or documentation about a patient's condition or treatment without consent. Personal information about the patient is considered protected health information (PHI), and it includes any identifying or personal information about the patient, such as health history,

- 34 -

condition, or treatments in any form, and any documentation. Failure to comply with HIPAA regulations can make a nurse liable for legal action.

14. C: Ego integrity vs. despair. Erikson's stages include the following:

Trust vs. mistrust	Birth to 1 year	Can result in mistrust or faith and optimism.
Autonomy vs. shame/doubt	1–3 years	Can lead to doubt and shame or self-control and willpower.
Initiative vs. guilt	3–6 years	Can lead to guilt or direction and purpose.
Industry vs. inferiority	6–12 years	Can lead to inadequacy and inferiority or competence.
Identity vs. role confusion	12–18 years	Can lead to role confusion or devotion and fidelity to others.
Intimacy vs. isolation	Young adulthood	Can lead to lack of close relationships or love/intimacy.
Generativity vs. stagnation	Middle age	Can lead to stagnation or caring and achievements.
Ego integrity vs. despair	Older adulthood	Can lead to despair (failure to accept changes of aging) or wisdom (acceptance).

15. A: Subjective notes usually quote what the client states directly: "I don't want to do this!" Objective notes record what is observed, clinical facts: "Patient sitting with arms folded, yawning frequently, and closing eyes." Assessment relates to evaluation of subjective and objective notes: "Patient appears tired. He has been complaining of insomnia." Plan is based on assessment: "Administer antidepressant in the morning rather than at bedtime and schedule a daily nap."

16. D: If a 52-year-old patient with heart disease is having difficulty with smoking cessation, the AGACNP should advise the patient that the most effective method of reducing the temptation to smoke is to avoid triggers. If, for example, the patient typically started each day with a cup of coffee, a newspaper, and a cigarette, the patient needs to alter this habit and omit the coffee or read the newspaper at a different time.

17. B: Gross negligence. Negligence indicates that *proper care* has not been provided, based on established standards. *Reasonable care* uses a rationale for decision-making in relation to providing care. Types of negligence include:

- Negligent conduct indicates that an individual failed to provide reasonable care or to protect/assist another, based on standards and expertise.
- Gross negligence is willfully providing inadequate care while disregarding the safety and security of another.
- Contributory negligence involves the injured party contributing to his/her own harm.
- Comparative negligence attempts to determine what percentage amount of negligence is attributed to each individual involved.

18. C: The most important consideration is the education and skills of the person to whom the task is delegated. The five rights of delegation include:

- Right task: Determine an appropriate task to delegate for a specific patient.
- Right circumstance: Consider the setting, resources, time factors, safety factors, and all other relevant information to determine the appropriateness of delegation.
- Right person: Choose the right person (by virtue of education/skills) to perform a task for the right patient.
- Right direction: Provide a clear description of the task, the purpose, any limits, and expected outcomes.
- Right supervision: Supervise, intervene as needed, and evaluate performance of the task.

19. D: Prealbumin (transthyretin) is most commonly monitored for acute changes in nutritional status because it has a half-life of only 2–3 days.

Mild deficiency: 10–15mg/dL.

Moderate deficiency: 5–9 mg/dL.

Severe deficiency: <5 mg/dL.

Prealbumin is a good measurement because it quickly decreases when nutrition is inadequate and rises quickly in response to increased protein intake. Protein intake must be adequate to maintain levels of prealbumin. Total protein and transferrin levels can be influenced by many factors. Albumin has a half-life of 18–20 days, so it is more sensitive to long-term protein deficiencies than to short-term protein deficiencies.

20. B: Left-hemisphere strokes are characterized by right-sided paresis/paralysis, short-term memory loss, depression, right visual field defect, and aphasia. Right-hemisphere strokes result in left paralysis or paresis and a left visual field deficit. Fine motor skills may be impacted, resulting in trouble with dressing. People may become impulsive, depressed, and exhibit poor judgment, often denying impairment, and may have short-term memory loss, but language remains intact. Brain stem strokes may involve motor and/or sensory impairment and respiratory and cardiac abnormalities. Cerebellar strokes may result in ataxia, nausea and vomiting, headaches, and dizziness or vertigo.

21. A: When assessing a patient with a history of alcohol abuse, the laboratory study that is especially important to include is liver function tests because alcohol abuse puts the patient at risk for development of cirrhosis as well as hepatic carcinoma. The patient should also have a complete blood count (CBC) with differential, comprehensive metabolic panel, and amylase and lipase tests because of the increased risk for pancreatitis. Some patients may also require screening tests for other abused substances.

22. D: If a 15-year-old patient reports that an adult touched her "private parts" against the patient's wishes, the most appropriate statement or question by the AGACNP is "What specific part of your body do you mean when you say 'private parts'?" It's important to clarify. If the patient is reluctant to respond, offering multiple choices ("your breasts?" "your vagina?" "your face?") is less leading than giving only one choice.

23. B: The tracer methodology looks at the continuum of care a patient receives from admission to post discharge. A patient is selected to be "traced," and the medical record serves as a guide. Tracer methodology uses the experience of this patient to evaluate the processes in place through

documents and interviews. Root cause analysis (RCA) is a retrospective attempt to determine the cause of an event, often a sentinel event such as an unexpected death, or a cluster of events. Root cause analysis involves interviews, observations, and review of medical records. Family and staff surveys may provide helpful but less detailed information.

24. D: The greatest risk factor for the development of methicillin-resistant *Staphylococcus aureus* (MRSA) pneumonia is intubation and ventilation, especially in intensive care units, possibly because patients have multiple risk factors. The risk of developing infection is about 1 to 3% for each day of intubation. Pneumonia that occurs on days 1 to 4 is usually antibiotic sensitive, but later onset pneumonia is often resistant. Treatment for MRSA pneumonia is with vancomycin or linezolid for 1 to 3 weeks.

25. A: Distribution of drugs is often impaired in gerontological patients because of changes in body water volume. Body water volume tends to decrease at the same time that fat deposits increase and are distributed differently. These changes especially affect the distribution of lipophilic drugs and may also increase their half-lives. Distribution may also be affected by decreased levels of albumin, which decreases plasma protein binding.

26. C: If a patient is diagnosed with Parkinson's disease but symptoms are very mild, levodopa is often withheld until symptoms worsen because the drug's effectiveness decreases over time. Levodopa is usually given with carbidopa to relieve nausea and other adverse effects. (The combination drug is Sinemet). Some drugs, such as tolcapone and entacapone, prolong the effectiveness of levodopa, so levodopa can be given earlier in treatment.

27. B: A pH level of >7 (alkaline) of aspirant from a nasogastric tube most likely indicates that the tube tip is in the respiratory system. Gastric fluids tend to be acidic (although this can be altered by medications), so pH usually ranges from 1 to 4. The pH in intestinal fluids is less acidic and should be approximately 6 or higher. Some tubes have pH sensors in place and do not require aspiration to check. Checking pH is not effective with continuous feedings because tube feedings usually have pH of 6.6 and have a neutralizing effect on gastrointestinal pH.

28. D: A patient who has been stable on medications for gastric ulcer and begins to complain of increasing back and epigastric pain unrelieved by medication may be experiencing erosion of the ulcer through the gastric serosa and into the surrounding organs and tissues, such as the pancreas or biliary tract. Penetration has a less acute presentation than perforation, which usually involves sudden acute abdominal pain (sometimes referred to the right shoulder), hypotension, bradycardia, omitting, and abdominal distension and rigidity.

29. C: When measuring the ankle-brachial index (ABI), the blood pressure cuff should be pumped 20 mm Hg higher than the pressure at which the last sound was heard on the Doppler ultrasound. The ABI is assessed with the patient lying supine. The arms are assessed one at a time with the Doppler over the brachial artery. The ankles are assessed with the Doppler over the posterior tibial pulse (the medial aspect of the ankle). Each ankle systolic pressure is divided by the brachial pressure to find the ABI. Normal values are 1 to 1.1. An ABI reading of <0.9 indicates arterial insufficiency.

30. A: The indication that a patient with diabetes has developed Charcot foot is when the foot takes on a rocker-bottom-shaped appearance. Charcot foot occurs when the bones weaken and fracture. It is associated with severe neuropathy and lack of sensation, so the patient continues to walk on the foot, resulting in the deformity. Treatment may include immobilization, custom shoes/braces, and activity limitation. Some patients require surgical repair.

31. B: If a 60-year-old male patient has mild prostatic hypertrophy with no urinary retention, the treatment of choice is likely watch and wait. There are adverse effects associated with all treatments, including the possibility of erectile dysfunction. Additionally, symptoms may subside in as many as 55% of patients without treatment. However, if symptoms progress, then a more aggressive approach may be considered, including alpha-blockers, 5 alpha-reductase inhibitors, phosphodiesterase-5 inhibitor, phytotherapy (plant-based), and various surgical options.

32. D: Although trends will show some normal variation, if the trend becomes erratic and measures are inconsistent, this suggests that the processes of care are not consistent or are inadequate. Tracking and trending are central to developing research-supported, evidence-based practice, and they are a part of continuous quality improvement. Once processes and outcomes measurements are selected, then at least one measure should be tracked for a number of periods of time, usually in increments of 4 weeks or quarterly. This tracking can be used to present graphical representation of results that will show trends.

33. C: A low-fat diet is usually recommended for those with chronic pancreatitis. Because the production of pancreatic enzymes may be impaired, patients may also need to take pancreatic enzymes with meals. If insulin production is affected, then some patients may require treatment for diabetes with insulin and diet modified to restrict carbohydrates. Because about 45% of those with chronic pancreatitis suffer from alcohol abuse, restricting alcohol intake is critical, so some patients may require referral to substance abuse programs.

34. B: Total parenteral nutrition (TPN) is high in glucose, so patients should have blood glucose levels monitored every 6 hours to evaluate hyperglycemia. Some patients may require insulin during administration of parenteral nutrition. Symptoms of hyperglycemia may include increased thirst, increased urination, blurred vision, and lethargy. Some patients may experience a rebound hypoglycemia when TPN is discontinued. The goal of TPN is usually for the patient to gain about 0.5 kg daily. Once the patient's symptoms decrease and weight stabilizes, the patient is placed on oral elemental feedings.

35. A: If a 28-year-old patient with three young children has ovarian cancer and is to be discharged to her home with fentanyl transdermal patches for pain control, when teaching the patient about the use of the patches, the AGACNP should stress that discarded patches must be folded and immediately flushed down the toilet. Used patches still contain the opioid and can result in the overdose and death of small children who come in contact with them and are a grave risk to drug seekers who smoke discarded patches.

36. B: If a 26-year-old patient presents with a rapidly developing sore throat that is severely painful, especially when attempting to swallow, and she is sitting in tripod position with the mouth open and drooling, these signs and symptoms are characteristic of epiglottitis, in which the epiglottis swells and can block the airway. Treatment includes immediate hospitalization for IV antibiotics (ceftizoxime or cefuroxime) and corticosteroids (dexamethasone). Some patients (10%) will require intubation and ventilation.

37. D: The most common cause of distributive shock is sepsis (septic shock). With distributive shock, arterial/venous dilation occurs, resulting in decreased systemic vascular resistance and decreased cardiac output and tissue hypoperfusion, although blood volume is normal. Sepsis usually develops from bacteremia. Common causes include *Escherichia coli, Klebsiella, Proteus,* and *Pseudomonas.* Risk factors include older age, diabetes, recent invasive procedures, and immunosuppression. Distributive shock may occur with sepsis, anaphylaxis, neurological insult, vasodilator drugs, and acute adrenal insufficiency.

38. A: If the AGACNP is conducting clinical research and intends to select participants that will be able to provide a particular perspective related to the research question, this is an example of purposeful sampling because selection is based on the needs of the study. Nominated sampling enrolls participants through recommendations of those already enrolled. Convenience or volunteer sampling requires finding participants through solicitation or advertising. Theoretical sampling is a form of purposeful sample that uses participants to build a theory.

39. C: If a patient was recently divorced and makes the negative statement, "I can't manage on my own," the most therapeutic response in helping the patient cope with this stressful situation is "Can you think of something positive about being on your own?" Thinking positively can be difficult for patients, especially those who tend to be pessimistic, but when patients make negative statements, they should be encouraged to counter that with a positive statement.

40. D: If a 49-year-old male complains of severe chest pain radiating to left shoulder and arm, and vital signs include BP, 152/92; P, 96; R, 20; oxygen saturation, 94%; temperature, 38°C (100.4°F); the patient is nauseated; the skin is clammy; and ECG shows anterior STEMI, the treatment priority should include acetylsalicylic acid (ASA) 324 mg and a nitrate sublingually every 5 minutes as needed for up to 15 minutes. If the nitrate is ineffective in relieving pain, then morphine should be administered. Oxygen may be necessary, although oxygen saturation at 94% is only slightly outside normal parameters (95% to 100%).

41. B: A realistic goal to be included in the care plan of a patient with diabetes mellitus is an A1c level of less than 7%. Other goals should include maintaining a preprandial glucose level of 70 to 130 mg/dL (3.9 to 7.2 mmol/L) and a peak postprandial glucose level of less than 180 mg/dL (10 mmol/L). Although these goals are ideal, they may need to be modified for the individual patient, depending on the severity of diabetes, comorbidities, age, and other factors.

42. C: Low-dose inhaled corticosteroid.

Asthma treatment for intermittent asthma and exacerbations		
Step	**Recommendation**	**Alternatives**
Step 1	Short-acting beta-2 agonist (SABA)	—
Step 2	Low-dose inhaled corticosteroid (ICS)	Cromolyn, leukotriene receptor antagonist (LTRA), nedocromil, or theophylline.
Step 3	Low-dose ICS plus long-acting beta-2 agonist (LABA)	Low-dose ICS plus LTRA, theophylline, or zileuton.
Step 4	Medium-dose ICS plus LABA	Low-dose ICS plus LTRA, theophylline, or zileuton.
Step 5	High-dose ICS plus LABA	Consider omalizumab with allergies.
Step 6	High-dose ICS plus LABA plus oral corticosteroid	Consider omalizumab with allergies.

43. A: If a patient being treated for endocarditis has developed sudden onset of hematuria, the AGACNP should suspect possible renal embolization. Embolization is a great risk during the first 3 months of treatment and may result in stroke, pulmonary embolus, and splenic embolization as well as renal embolization. Endocarditis can result from transient or chronic bacteremia, and it may occur in patients who are IV drug users or those with prosthetic heart disease, rheumatic heart disease, mitral valve prolapse, and other cardiac abnormalities.

44. D: If a 78-year-old patient with COPD is hospitalized with acute respiratory distress syndrome (ARDS), pronounced wheezing, fever (38.6°C [101.5°F]), and cough; the arterial blood gases are pH, 7.24; paO_2, 49 mm Hg; $paCO_2$, 61 mm Hg; the patient is provided steroids and bronchodilators; and is alert and able to follow directions but unable to speak because of dyspnea, the treatment that is most appropriate to relieve respiratory distress is noninvasive ventilation (NIV). NIV does not require intubation.

45. A: If the AGACNP works with a group of ethnically diverse staff members, but a number of conflicts have arisen because of different methods of communication and attitudes toward authority, the best solution is likely to initiate a discussion about cultural differences, including direct versus indirect communication. Ignoring the situation or issuing guidelines is not likely to alter the situation unless the problem is dealt with directly by those involved. Through discussion, better approaches to communication may develop.

46. C: If a patient is receiving methotrexate for maintenance treatment of Crohn's disease, laboratory tests that should be routinely monitored include the complete blood count (CBC) and renal function (creatinine and BUN) and liver function tests. Food and Drug Administration (FDA) guidelines advise testing at least every 1 to 2 months during therapy, but some authorities recommend testing every 2 to 4 weeks during the first few months of treatment. Adverse effects of methotrexate include renal failure, portal fibrosis, myelosuppression, headache, and rash.

47. B: If a 19-year-old female patient with sickle cell disease experienced an aplastic crisis with hemoglobin of 5.6 g/dL (56 mmol/L), the patient will likely receive transfusions of packed red blood cells until the patient's hemoglobin reaches 10 g/dL (100 mmol/L). Hemoglobin levels of 6 to 9 g/dL (60 to 90 mmol/L) are common in patients with sickle cell disease because their red blood cells (RBCs) survive only 10 to 12 days rather than the normal 120 days.

48. D: If a patient who was a victim of a violent assault and rape is shaking and crying and appears terrified, the most therapeutic response at the time of the initial encounter with the patient is "You are safe now." The patient is likely still in the "fight-or-flight" mode with increased adrenalin from having to deal with the assault and rape, police intervention, and now a medical examination, so it's important for the AGACNP to provide calm reassurance to the patient to try to allay fears.

49. A: If the AGACNP examines a patient's functional ability and notes that his gait is characterized by shuffling of the feet with periodic short, rapid steps while the neck, trunk, and knees are flexed and the patient is leaning forward, increasingly walking faster, the AGACNP should recognize this gait as being characteristic of Parkinson's disease. The patient may also exhibit a blank facial expression; slow, monotonous, or slurred speech; and tremors. Classic manifestations include the triad of tremor, rigidity, and bradykinesia.

50. C: If a 60-year-old patient's BP ranges from 140–159/90–99, the BP is classified as stage 1 hypertension.

BP classification	
Normal	<120/<80
Prehypertension	120–139/80–89
Stage 1 hypertension	140–159/90–99
Stage 2 hypertension	≥160/≥100

Lifestyle modifications (decrease alcohol, stop smoking, lose weight, increase exercise, and reduce stress) is encouraged for those with high BP and strongly recommended for all others.

51. B: If an 86-year-old patient has developed painful lesions extending from the left side of her back around to the left side of her chest, indicating probable herpes zoster (shingles) infection, the most appropriate treatment is an antiviral (such as acyclovir, famciclovir, or valacyclovir). Although this will not cure the infection, it may reduce the severity. If pain is severe, the patient may also require analgesia. Cool compresses may relieve discomfort and itching. Some patients may develop postherpetic neuralgia with severe pain that may last for weeks, months, or indefinitely.

52. C: If a patient under hospice care for end-of-life care for stage 4 multiple myeloma has developed severe skeletal pain and is scheduled to undergo radiation therapy to reduce discomfort, this treatment does not affect hospice care because—although radiation may be an active treatment in some cases—the intent of the treatment is to provide palliation rather than to delay disease progress or to cure the disease. Although there is no preauthorization process for treatment under hospice, there are appeal processes that are available if hospice service has been denied.

53. D: The patient most at risk for development of a chronic subdural hematoma 3 to 4 weeks after initial injury is the 78-year-old patient who fell and hit his head on the floor but experienced only a slight headache at the time. Chronic subdural hematomas are most common in the elderly, probably because atrophy of the brain allows for more movement during injury, which can tear vessels. In many cases of subdural hematoma, patients do not recall any prior injury.

54. A: If a patient developed SIADH after taking sertraline, which is associated with hyponatremia, and the patient's serum sodium level was 120mEq/L (120 mmol/L), and the patient exhibited mild confusion, anorexia, and nausea, in addition to discontinuation of the sertraline, the first-line intervention is to limit fluid intake. Severe neurological damage can occur if the sodium level is increased too rapidly, so the patient must be carefully monitored. Normal values for serum sodium are 135 to 145 mEq/L (135 to 145 mmol/L) with hyponatremia of less than 120 mEq/L (120 mmol/L) being a critical finding.

55. B: If a patient with end-stage renal disease develops a hypertensive crisis with BP of 182/108, heart rate of 104 beats per minute, respirations of 18 per minute, and oxygen saturation of 98% and the patient is anxious and complains of headache but there is no indication of organ damage, this type of hypertensive crisis is categorized as a hypertensive urgency. The patient must be monitored closely while receiving labetalol because the blood pressure must be reduced slowly to avoid hypotension and ischemia of internal organs. Reduction should be about 33% in the first 6 hours, 33% in the next 24 hours, and 33% over the next 2 to 4 days.

56. A: If a 64-year-old male African-American patient with diabetes has BP readings that average about 154/96, the first-line pharmacologic therapy that the AGACNP should advise is a thiazide diuretic or calcium channel blocker. If a patient is of a different ethnic group, the initial therapy may include a thiazide diuretic, calcium channel blocker, ACE inhibitor, or ARB. If the patient does not respond adequately to the first drug, most often a thiazide diuretic, then a second drug and, in some cases, a third drug can be added. ACE inhibitors should not be given with ARBs.

57. C: If a 28-year-old female patient is recovering from a Zika infection and tells the AGACNP that she has been trying to conceive, the patient should be advised to wait for at least 8 weeks to try again to conceive, according to CDC guidelines. However, if the male partner has been possibly exposed, they should wait for at least 6 months after possible exposure or symptoms begin and should have only protected sex.

58. D: If a Navajo patient tells the AGACNP that he has "ghost sickness," the most appropriate response is: "How does ghost sickness make you feel?" This response respects the patient's

perception of the disease and helps the nurse to understand what symptoms the patient is attributing to the disorder. The Navajo believe that ghost sickness is brought about by evil spirits, and they believe that a tribal healer may be able to overcome the spirit. Typical symptoms include weakness, nightmares, fear, and feelings of suffocation.

59. B: If a patient with hypertrophic cardiomyopathy has been prescribed propranolol, the AGACNP should inform the patient and family members that patients taking the drug are at risk for depression, affecting 50% or more, especially those with a history of depression or substance abuse. The patient should be aware of the signs and symptoms of depression and should notify the AGACNP if they occur. The patient should be advised to never abruptly stop the drug because doing so could cause a myocardial infarction or cardiac arrest.

60. A: If a patient in good health had a sudden onset of weakness, chest pain, and dyspnea with systolic BP palpable at 52 mm Hg, pulse 128, R 38, and oxygen saturation of 81% on room air, then the test that may be used to rule out pulmonary embolism is the D-dimer assay. If the test is negative, then pulmonary embolism is unlikely. If, however, it is positive, then imaging such as CT scan or pulmonary angiography should be carried out. Arterial blood gases, although not diagnostic for pulmonary embolism, should be performed to determine the patient's acid-base status.

61. D: If a patient is diagnosed with tuberculosis and must take antituberculosis drugs, taking methadone for heroin addiction may be an indication for directly observed therapy (DOT). With DOT, a healthcare worker administers each dose and observes the patient taking the medication to ensure that the treatment regimen is followed. Other indications include multidrug-resistant tuberculosis (MDR-TB) and extensively drug resistant TB (XDR-TB), sputum cultures positive for acid-fast bacilli, psychiatric disease or cognitive impairment, homelessness, and demonstrated lack of adherence to treatment.

62. C: If the AGACNP notes that staffing patterns do not always match the workload in the acute care unit, the first step to a solution is to determine how staffing decisions are made. The AGACNP should always take action based on relevant information and data and should try to understand the views of management, his or her own personal views, and staff views in order to identify areas of agreement and possible compromise before researching staffing alternate methods and making suggestions for change.

63. B: Symptoms of cholecystitis include upper abdominal pain, sometimes localizing to the right upper quadrant (RUQ), fever, and nausea and vomiting, but these symptoms are nonspecific and may be found with acute gastritis, appendicitis, acute pyelonephritis, and other conditions of the gallbladder such as cancer. An ultrasound is usually done to confirm the presence of gallstones and blockage. Although conservative treatment may be effective in uncomplicated cases, most patients are referred for surgical intervention.

64. A: Scant tissue loss: Partial thickness injury and ≤25% of the epidermal flap lost.

The following table details the Payne-Martin classification for skin tears:

Payne-Martin classification for skin tears	
Category I Skin tear without tissue loss	*Linear: Full-thickness wound in a wrinkle or furrow with the epidermis and dermis pulled apart (incisional appearance). *Flap: Partial-thickness wound with a flap that can cover the wound with $\leq$ 1 mm of dermis exposed.
Category II Skin tear with partial tissue loss	*Scant tissue loss: Partial-thickness injury and $\leq$25% of epidermal flap lost. *Moderate to large tissue loss: Partial-thickness injury with >25% epidermal flap lost.
Category III Skin tear with complete tissue loss	*Complete partial-thickness injury with loss of epidermal flap.

65. D: If the AGACNP observes an unlicensed assistive personnel (UAP) massaging the reddened heels of an immobile patient, the AGACNP should explain how massaging reddened tissue may cause tissue damage. This was at one time a common practice, so the AGACNP should use this opportunity to update the UAP on evidence-based skin care guidelines and should provide guidance to the UAP regarding measures to relieve pressure, including the use of heel protectors, positioning, and frequent turning.

66. D: If the hospital administration has collected patient surveys to determine the needs that patients feel are most important, the next step in the quality improvement process should be to assemble a multidisciplinary team to review the results of the survey. Next, the team should collect data about the current status of these needs and determine measurable outcomes and quality indicators. Then, the team should select a plan, implement the plan, and collect data to evaluate outcomes.

67. B: If the AGACNP discovers that a patient faces various problems in returning home after discharge, including lack of adequate income and impaired ability to prepare food, and refers the patient to a social worker for assistance, the type of power that the AGACNP is exhibiting is advocacy power because the AGACNP is assisting the patient to overcome obstacles. Integrative power helps the patient return to normal life. Transformational power helps patients transform their self-image. Affirmative power is the strength the AGACNP gains from caring for patients.

68. A: If, when reviewing staffing needs, the AGACNP finds that staff members' time is most impacted by answering patients' call lights and responding to their needs, the strategy that is likely to be most effective for time saving is rounding on patients hourly. Rounding involves actually visiting each patient briefly to ask about and attend to needs, such as for pain control or toileting. Studies indicate that hourly rounding decreases call lights, falls, and pressure sores and increases patient satisfaction.

69. C: If a patient who developed polyarthralgia was recently diagnosed with systemic lupus erythematosus, when educating the patient about lifestyle changes, the AGACNP should plan to include energy conservation and skin protection. Fatigue is a chronic problem, so the patient must learn to pace activities and schedule periods of rest. Patients must ensure skin integrity by avoiding exposure to the sun, inspecting skin routinely, and using sunscreens. Patients also require education regarding management of chronic pain through analgesic and nonanalgesic means.

70. A: If an 18-year-old football player experienced blunt trauma to his lower left leg during a tackle and was able to walk initially with no difficulty but comes to the hospital about an hour later complaining of severe pain and tightness in the lower leg as well as a sensation of burning, and the lower leg is edematous and the skin is taut although a distal pulse is palpable and the capillary refill time is within normal limits, the priority intervention should be to measure compartment pressure to confirm compartment syndrome. Distal pulses and capillary refill time may remain intact until the damage is irreversible.

71. D: If the AGACNP is caring for a patient with kidney failure and a falling glomerular filtration rate (GFR) of 28 mL/min/1.73^2, the AGACNP should recognize that the patient is at stage 3 and will need renal replacement therapy when the GFR is less than 15 ml/min/1.73^2. The five stages of chronic kidney disease are listed as follows:

Stage 1: GFR >90 mL/min/1.73m^2. Usually asymptomatic.

Stage 2: GFR 60 to 89 mL/min/1.73m^2. Mild anemia/electrolyte imbalances.

Stage 3: GFR 30 to 59 mL/min/1.73m^2. Increasing fatigue, anemia, fluid retention, and blood pressure.

Stage 4: GFR 15 to 29 mL/min/1.73m^2. Profound disease.

Stage 5: GFR <15 mL/min/1.73m^2. Kidney failure.

72. D: If a patient who experienced tonic-clonic seizures is newly diagnosed with epilepsy and has started on antiseizure medication, when the AGACNP is educating the patient about the disease, the most important advice is to never stop taking the medication abruptly because this can trigger status epilepticus, which is life threatening. The patient should be advised to consult a healthcare provider if he or she is unable to take medication for any reason, such as illness. The patient should exercise in moderation and avoid excessive heat and should try to distinguish triggers and auras related to seizures to better manage the disorder.

73. B: Oxygen exchange in the lungs decreases with age because of enlargement of alveoli and alveolar ducts. Although the number of alveoli usually stays about the same, the enlargement results from loss of elastic fibers around the alveoli and ducts. Although these changes usually result in no overt symptoms, the decrease in air exchange may make older adults less tolerant to exercise, and some may find that they become "winded" more easily. Other changes include decreased glandular epithelial cells (reducing the production of mucus), and loss of elastin and collagen (allowing airways to collapse during expiration).

74. D: Confirmability. In evaluating research as part of the development of evidence-based practice guidelines, the four evaluative/trustworthiness criteria are listed as follows:

Credibility: Documentation supports accuracy and validity.

Dependability: Evidence shows how conclusion are reached and whether others should expect to reach the same conclusions.

Transferability: The extent to which the results can apply to others in similar situations.

Confirmability: The data are clear and show how conclusions are reached.

75. C: If a 66-year-old male patient complains of increasing abdominal pain and has been passing 3 to 4 sticky, black, foul-smelling stools for 3 to 4 days, his vital signs are BP, 116/78 supine; P, 112; R, 22; temperature, 37°C (98.6°F), his standing BP drops to 88/58 with dizziness, and the patient's hemoglobin is 9.2 mg/dL (92 mmol/L), hematocrit is 28%, mean cell volume (MCV) is 70 fL, and BUN is 46 mg/dL (16.4 mmol/L), the AGACNP should suspect iron deficiency anemia with upper GI bleeding. The anemia occurs from blood loss (low hemoglobin and hematocrit resulting in low MCV) and the melena is from blood in the upper GI tract that is exposed to digestive enzymes. The elevated BUN reflects the absorption of blood.

76. A: If a 30-year-old male patient is to be discharged after a vasectomy, when educating the patient, the AGACNP should stress the importance of using an alternate form of contraception, such as a condom, for 6 to 8 weeks because sperm may remain alive for months within the semen. The patient should be advised to return for postoperative sperm count at 3 months or after 20 to 25 ejaculations.

77. D: If a patient recently returned from serving in the military in the Middle East is hospitalized with post-traumatic stress disorder (PTSD) and the patient has recurring flashbacks and nightmares and is constantly vigilant and anxious, telling the AGACNP repeatedly that he should have died with his friends, the most appropriate response is: "Are you thinking about killing yourself?" When a patient gives clues about suicidal ideation, it is the AGACNP's responsibility to address the issue with the patient, and patients often want to talk about their feelings.

78. B: If the AGACNP is screening patients for referral to a case manager, the patient that is most likely to benefit from case management is the 62-year-old patient with repeated hospitalizations from chronic obstructive pulmonary disease (COPD) and diabetes. Criteria for case management include patients with severe chronic illness and comorbidities, especially those with a history of repeated hospitalizations or noncompliance with treatment and those who are elderly, disabled, or impaired and lack an adequate support system.

79. B: If a patient with dilated cardiomyopathy is on the transplant list for a heart but none has become available, the patient's ejection fraction has fallen to 22%, and the patient's functional ability is markedly decreased, the AGACNP should recognize that the patient may benefit most from a left ventricular assist device (LVAD). The LVAD is usually implanted in patients whose ejection fraction is less than 25% (normal values range from 55 to 65%). The LVAD augments the heart's ability to pump blood and can be used as a bridge to transplant or as destination treatment for those who are not candidates for transplant.

80. A: If a patient with chronic low back pain states that he wants to try complementary therapy to relive pain because medications have been ineffective and asks the AGACNP which of the therapies are likely to relieve discomfort, the AGACNP should reply that the therapy that has documented effectiveness is acupuncture. Acupuncture appears to stimulate the production of endorphins. Acupuncture is generally safe and has no adverse effects if done by an experienced practitioner. There is little discomfort involved in treatment.

81. D: If a patient scheduled for removal of a colon tumor and creation of a colostomy asks about whether stools will be regular after surgery, the AGACNP should advise the patient that bowel regularity can be expected if the tumor is in the descending colon or rectum because stool is formed. Fecal output may be controlled with daily irrigations and a small pouch or dressing over the stoma. Higher in the colon, the stool is more liquid and may drain more freely, requiring constant use of colostomy bags.

82. B: <u>Privileging</u> follows the credentialing process and grants the individual authority to practice within the organization. <u>Credentialing</u> is the process by which a person's credentials to provide patient care are obtained, verified, and assessed in accordance with organizational bylaws, which may vary from one organization to another. Decisions regarding credentialing and privileging are usually done by members of a credentials committee, although some organizations use Internet services to verify credentials. Part of credentialing and privileging is to determine what credentials are necessary for different positions, based on professional standards, licensure, regulatory guidelines, and accreditation guidelines.

83. C: The primary criterion for referral to a hospice program is the probability that death will occur within 6 months. Generally, hospice programs require a do-not-resuscitate (DNR) order and a diagnosis of a life-threatening disease, but those alone are not sufficient, because patients with longer life expectancies should be referred to palliative care programs instead. Severe intractable pain may be one problem hospice addresses, but pain can occur in patients who do not have a life-threatening disease.

84. D: A <u>court order</u> authorizes disclosure of a patient's personal health information. In some cases, this court order may cover only restricted information rather than an entire health record. A <u>subpoena</u> is issued to advise a person that he or she must give testimony in court or in a deposition. A <u>subpoena duces tecum</u> is similar but requires the person to bring specific documents to court. A <u>warrant</u> authorizes an action, such as a search.

85. A: Collaboration is an essential element when the AGACNP is using adult learning principles to work with adult learners. The adult must be an active participant in establishing learning goals and determining their own learning experiences. Although adults tend to be self-directed, not all adults feel comfortable applying this self-direction to education, so the AGACNP must provide guidance to allay the fear of failure that is also common among adults. The primary role of the AGACNP is that of facilitator.

86. C: The most effective method to ensure that team members in an acute care unit are prepared to carry out the disaster plan in case of emergency is to schedule practice/simulation drills. Simulations may include fire drills to determine if the staff knows how to protect patients, contain small blazes, and evacuate. More extensive simulations may include various scenarios with volunteer "patients" and simulated injuries. Prior to the simulations, the staff members should be educated about the disaster plan and should review established protocols.

87. B: A patient with schizophrenia should be evaluated for the common comorbidities of depression, obsessive-compulsive disorder, panic disorders, and suicidal ideation. Additionally, most (up to 90%) are heavy smokers and many self-medicate with alcohol and drugs. Patients with schizophrenia have high rates of diabetes and heart disease, often undiagnosed and untreated, especially for those who are homeless. Treatment does not cure schizophrenia but can make it manageable, although rates of nonadherence are very high, and about 30% do not respond adequately to antipsychotic drugs.

88. C: If a nonverbal young adult patient with autism spectrum disorder is scheduled for a minor surgical procedure and is accompanied by a parent, but the patient is very frightened, distressed, and uncooperative, the best way to reduce the patient's anxiety is to ask the parent for advice about appropriate interventions. The parent likely knows what triggers the patient's anxiety and what has a calming effect. Generally, touching a patient with autism spectrum disorder without asking first can be very distressing to him or her.

- 46 -

89. D: If a 59-year-old patient is admitted to the medical-surgical unit with pneumonia, acute hospitalization for 4 days 65 days (up to 90 days) previously is a risk factor for the development of healthcare-associated pneumonia. Other risk factors include the following:

- Acute hospitalization of ≥2 days within the previous 90 days.
- Long-term home dialysis within the previous 30 days.
- Residence in a long-term-care facility.
- Home infusion therapy within the previous 30 days.
- Antibiotic therapy within the previous 90 days.
- Home wound care.
- Family member with a multidrug-resistant infection.
- Immunosuppressive disease or therapy.

90. A: When determining the level of risk for evaluation and management (E/M) services, the three components of the Centers for Medicare & Medicaid Services (CMS) Table of Risk that must be considered are the presenting problem(s), diagnostic procedure(s) ordered, and management options selected. The table is used to determine the level of risk of complications, morbidity, and/or mortality: minimal, low, moderate, or high. The overall level of risk is determined by the highest level of risk in any of the three components.

91. C: The coding system that is used to code for outpatient diagnoses is ICD-10-CM. The same coding system is used to code for inpatient diagnoses as well, so there is consistency when patients transfer from one level of care to another. ICD-10-CM replaced ICD-9 in October 2015. Inpatient and outpatient services, however, use different coding systems for procedures. Inpatient facilities use ICD-10-PCS, and outpatient facilities use HCPCS/CPT. HCPCS level I codes incorporate the CPT codes, but level II codes are used for services not included as part of the CPT codes, such as ambulance service.

92. B: If a patient is brought to the emergency department after a motorcycle accident and exhibits bruising over the area of the mastoid process (Battle's sign) as well as otorrhea, these are indications of a basilar skull fracture. Rhinorrhea (clear cerebrospinal fluid [CSF]) and bilateral swelling and ecchymosis of the eyes (raccoon eyes) can also indicate a basilar skull fracture. Basilar skull fractures may occur from impacts to the occipital or mandibular areas and may result in damage to the olfactory and optic nerves.

93. C: Risk factors commonly associated with development of diabetes mellitus, type 2, include obesity and inactivity. Risk also increases with a family history of diabetes. Risk increases with age, possibly because of the tendency to gain weight and exercise less, although dietary changes have resulted in a substantial increase in the rates of diabetes among children and adolescents. Diet may increase risk, especially a diet high in simple carbohydrates, and diabetes risk increases with high levels of triglycerides (which reflect carbohydrate intake).

94. D: A male patient is considered at high risk for health problems if his waist-to-hip ratio is greater than 1.0. The waist-to-hip ratio risk is outlined as follows:

Gender	Ideal	Increased risk	High risk
Male	0.9 to 0.95	0.96 to 1.0	>1.0
Female	0.7 to 0.8	0.81 to 0.85	>0.85

Body shape is often described as "pear" or "apple," and apple-shaped individuals carry more fat in the abdomen, putting them at greater risk, especially for myocardial infarction (MI). The waist-to-hip ratio is a better predictor of MI than the BMI.

95. B: The fracture that is likely to result in the greatest loss of blood is the pelvis.

Estimated blood loss with fractures (in liters)	
Ankle	0.5 to 1.5
Elbow	0.5 to 1.5
Femur	1 to 2
Hip	1.5 to 2.5
Humerus	1 to 2
Knee	1 to 1.5
Pelvis	1.5 to 4.5
Tibia	0.5 to 1.5

96. C: If an older patient complains of urinary frequency and urgency, increasing shortness of breath, pain in the right knee when walking prolonged distances, and chronic constipation, the order of priority (most critical to least) should be:

1. Shortness of breath: Problems with airway breathing circulation (ABCs) have priority because they may be life threatening.
2. Urinary frequency and urgency: This may indicate or increase the risk of infection or renal problems.
3. Chronic constipation: This is an ongoing problem that requires intervention.
4. Pain in the right knee: Because this only occurs when walking prolonged distances, this problem has the lowest priority.

97. A: If an AGACNP copies and pastes free text from one patient's electronic health record to another when the information needed is similar, this is a dangerous practice. Documentation must be individualized for the patient and not copied from another patient. Even a small mistake may result in serious consequences for the patient's healthcare as well as for billing. The copy and paste function should only be used sparingly within a patient's electronic health record (EHR), such as copying and pasting a problem list or patient history to the patient's discharge summary.

98. C: Although shared governance focuses primarily on empowering nursing, partnership councils focus on members at all levels of an organization and all departments. Rather than one large partnership council, an organization may have a number of partnership councils with one member from each assigned to attend the central council. This prevents the central council from becoming too large to work effectively. Communication flows both vertically and horizontally, and information is shared throughout the organization.

99. C: If a 72-year-old patient complains of increasing fatigue, weakness, dyspnea on exertion, and lack of interest in activities, and the pulse rate increases from 70 to 96, blood pressure from 126/78 to 150/96, and respirations from 18 to 26 three minutes after activity, a likely nursing diagnosis is activity intolerance. The patient must be assessed for cardiovascular or other disorders that could be causing the activity intolerance and imbalance between the supply of oxygen and the demand. The condition can also result from a sedentary lifestyle or long periods of immobility or bedrest.

100. B: Patients who are taking phenytoin for seizure disorders should be advised to have regular dental care because of the increased risk of gingival hyperplasia, which can occur both in children

and adults and can lead to bleeding, tooth displacement, and periodontal disease. Phenytoin-induced gingival hyperplasia occurs in 15% to 50% of patients taking the medication. Poor oral hygiene is a risk factor, so patients on phenytoin should be educated about the need for regular dental care, brushing and flossing, as well as routine teeth cleaning and examinations by dentists.

101. A: When assessing for facial palsy as part of the National Institutes of Health (NIH) Stroke Scale, the part of the face that is the best place to focus on for minor paralysis is the mouth. For this section, the patient is asked to show teeth, raise eyebrows, and close eyes. Scoring is performed as follows:

> 0 = Normal symmetrical movements.
>
> 1 = Minor paralysis (flattened nasolabial fold, asymmetry on smiling).
>
> 2 = Partial paralysis (total or near-total paralysis of the lower face).
>
> 3 = Complete paralysis of one or both sides (absence of facial movement in the upper and lower face).

102. C: If, when the AGACNP is screening telephone calls in the acute care telehealth program, a patient calls to complain of low back pain, the additional symptoms that represent an emergent situation and should result in the nurse advising the patient to hang up and call 9-1-1 is sudden loss of bowel and bladder control. Pain radiating down the left leg may indicate pressure on the sciatic nerve, whereas fever or burning on urination and frequency may indicate a urinary tract infection. These conditions are not emergent, but appointments should be made as soon as possible.

103. C: An example of tertiary prevention for patients with diabetes mellitus is annual screening for kidney disease because diabetes is the leading cause of kidney failure and the need for dialysis and/or kidney transplant. Because diabetes is also a leading cause of blindness, patients should be screened every 12 to 24 months for retinopathy. Patients should be screened at each visit for complications of the lower extremities (impaired circulation, ulcerations, sores, calluses, abrasions, neuropathy) because diabetes is a major cause of amputations.

104. B: Hypoglycemia is a differential diagnosis that must be ruled out for a patient presenting with possible stroke because of a sudden onset of decreased level of consciousness and unilateral weakness. If the patient is hypoglycemic, the cause (preexisting diabetes, insulin reaction) must be determined and appropriate treatment must be provided. When glucose levels return to normal, the symptoms should subside. Patients with diabetes are at increased risk of stroke, and severe hypoglycemia can result in brain damage.

105. D: The primary purpose of conducting a problem-based assessment on a patient is to create a problem list based on a thorough exam and history. Once a list of problems is identified, then the problems are prioritized so that the most critical issues are dealt with first. One problem may involve a number of different physical and psychosocial elements. For example, poor nutrition may relate to the inability to physically prepare food, depression, inadequate resources to purchase nutritious food, and lack of transportation.

106. A: In a patient with onset of myasthenia gravis (MG) at age 38, the organ that probably triggered the autoimmune response is the thymus. Early-onset MG (prior to age 40) is characterized by thymic hyperplasia, and treatment usually involves surgical removal of the thymus. In late-onset MG (after age 40), the thymus is generally normal although it still may be

involved in the autoimmune process. Patients whose MG is caused by thymoma are usually in the 40- to 60-year-old range.

107. D: If the AGACNP is concerned that an older patient may be drinking excessively, the CAGE Assessment may be the most appropriate tool.

C	Cutting down	Do you think about trying to cut down on drinking?
A	Annoyed at criticism	Are people starting to criticize your drinking?
G	Guilty feeling	Do you feel guilty or try to hide your drinking?
E	Eye-opener	Do you increasingly need a drink earlier in the day?

"Yes" on one question suggests the possibility of a drinking problem, whereas "yes" on ≥2 indicates a drinking problem.

108. A: If, when using the Plan-Do-Study-Act (PDSA) method of continuous quality improvement, study of the outcomes of a trial indicates that the solution that was instituted was not effective, the next step is to return to the plan step in order to select a different solution. The PDSA method is described as follows:

- Plan: Define the problem, brainstorm, and collect data.
- Do: Generate solutions, choose one, and implement a trial.
- Study: Evaluate outcomes.
- Act: Identify changes needed for full implementation and continue to monitor.

109. B: Stroke volume is the volume of blood that is ejected from the heart with every contraction and is equal to the end-diastolic volume minus the end-systolic volume. The normal value is usually 55 to 100 mL. The end-diastolic volume is the volume of blood in filled ventricles. End-systolic volume is the volume of blood left in the ventricles after contraction. Cardiac output is the total volume of blood ejected from the heart in one minute: heart rate times stroke volume. The normal cardiac output is 4.9L/min.

110. A: The primary tests that screen for hepatitis include alanine transaminase (ALT) (normal 5–35 units) and aspartate transaminase (AST) (normal 10–40 units). These are liver enzymes that increase with inflammation and damage to hepatic cells. ALT is more specific than AST and it usually shows a higher increase. ALT may increase to 10 times normal with acute infection and 2 to 3 times normal with chronic infection, so ALT is used most often to monitor treatment. However, many drugs can affect ALT results, so medication reconciliation is essential.

111. C: When counseling a 26-year-old patient with condylomata acuminata (genital warts), the AGACNP notes that the treatment with the highest success rate is surgical excision. This treatment also has the lowest recurrence rate. The cure rate from initial excision ranges from 63% to 91%. No treatment provides a 100% cure rate, and many must have repeated painful treatments, so the AGACNP should refer the patient to a specialist with experience treating condylomata acuminata.

112. D: Lipid screening should be done every 5 years starting at age 20. If levels are high, then patients may have more frequent screening:

Low-density lipoprotein (LDL) cholesterol	<100	Optimal
	100–129	Near optimal
	130–159	Borderline high
	160–189	High
	≥190	Very high
Total cholesterol	<200	Optimal
	200–239	Borderline high
	≥240	High
High-density lipoprotein (HDL) cholesterol	<40	Low
	≥60	High
Triglycerides	<150	Normal
	150–199	Borderline high
	200–499	High
	≥500	Very high

113. C: The Beers Criteria (American Geriatric Society) lists drugs that are inappropriate for older adults. The Beers Criteria can be incorporated into clinical decision support systems so that alerts are issued if a medication or dosage is inappropriate for the patient. The Beers Criteria lists the organ system/therapeutic category of the drugs, the rationale for including the drugs on the list, the recommendations (conditions for avoidance and exceptions), the quality and strength of evidence, as well as references.

114. B: Smoking electronic cigarettes, which deliver nicotine in an aerosol vapor ("vaping"), increases the risk of developing oral cancer. The vapor contains various substances, such as silica and metal, that can be damaging to oral tissues. Electronic cigarettes damage the cells of the oral cavity, which can lead to increased risk of infection and cell changes. Although some people are advised to use electronic cigarettes in order to quit smoking tobacco cigarettes, this has not been approved by the Food and Drug Administration (FDA).

115. A: If a 36-year-old HIV-positive patient is being tested for tuberculosis (TB) with a tuberculin skin test, a positive reaction for an HIV patient is induration of ≥5 mm.

Tuberculin skin test reactions	
≥5 mm	For patients who are HIV-positive, immunocompromised, or have had recent contact with people infected with TB or a history of prior TB.
≥10 mm	High-risk patients: recent immigrants, HIV-negative drug users, lab personnel, high-risk living situations (prisons, long-term care facilities, homeless shelters), and patients with diseases that put them at increased risk (such as leukemia, kidney disease, gastrectomy, cancer). Infants/Children younger than 4 and adolescents exposed to high-risk adults.
≥15 mm	Normal for patients with no TB risk factors.

116. C: If an older female patient with moderately advanced dementia is cradling a doll and says, "This is my baby," and refuses to relinquish the doll for an examination, the most appropriate response is: "I won't bother your baby." The confusion associated with dementia is different from hallucinations or delusions experienced by those with mental illness, so arguing and trying to

correct or reason with the patient is usually not helpful and may lead to agitation and aggressive behavior.

117. D: S3 occurs after S2 in children and young adults, but it may indicate heart failure or left ventricular failure in older adults (heard with the patient lying on the left side). S4 occurs before S1 and occurs with ventricular hypertrophy, such as from coronary artery disease, hypertension, or aortic valve stenosis. Opening snap is an unusual high-pitched sound occurring after S2 with mitral valve stenosis from rheumatic heart disease. Ejection click is a brief, high-pitched sound occurring immediately after S1 with aortic valve stenosis. Friction rub is a harsh, grating sound heard in systole and diastole with pericarditis.

118. B: Pregabalin (Lyrica), which is an anticonvulsant commonly prescribed for fibromyalgia, is believed to decrease pain by reducing electrical activity associated with overactive nerve impulses. Patients are usually treated initially with 150 mg/day in two divided doses increasing to 300 mg (maximum 450 mg). Adverse effects include allergic response, suicidal ideation, panic attacks, peripheral edema, sleepiness, and dizziness. Adverse effects may worsen if taken with alcohol, so alcohol should be avoided. Patients should be cautioned not to stop the medication abruptly.

119. C: If a 42-year-old patient with chronic lymphocytic leukemia (CLL) has developed thrombocytopenia, the patient may exhibit petechiae, gingival bleeding, nasal bleeding, and increased menstrual flow when the count drops below 20,000. The ability of the blood to clot decreases with a count below 50,000. The patient is likely to develop central nervous system (CNS) or gastrointestinal (GI) hemorrhage if the platelet count drops below 5000. Thrombocytopenia may result from decreased production of platelets in the bone marrow or increased destruction from the disease process or chemotherapy.

120. D: Variant (Prinzmetal's) angina results from spasms of the coronary arteries and is often related to smoking, alcohol, or illicit stimulants. Variant angina frequently occurs cyclically at the same time each day and often while the person is at rest. Stable angina episodes usually last for <5 minutes and are fairly predictable exercise-induced episodes caused by atherosclerotic lesions blocking >75% of the lumen of the effected coronary artery. Unstable angina is a progression of coronary artery disease and occurs with a change in the pattern of stable angina. Esophageal varices usually cause no symptoms before bleeding.

121. B: All members of the interdisciplinary team (IDT) should be involved in development of the plan of care and in major changes in the plan of care, but individual members of the team may assume responsibility for more specific matters, such as titrating pain medication, skin care, and stress reduction, in which they are directly involved. In many cases, the leader of the IDT is a physician, but decision-making should be a shared exercise. Nurses who provide direct care may have more insight into patient needs than other healthcare providers with less direct contact.

122. B: A full-thickness ulcer that extends to the tendon or joint but without abscess or osteomyelitis is classified as grade 2. The modified Wagner foot ulcer classification system separates foot ulcers into six grades (grade 0 to grade 5). Classification is based on depth of the lesion and the presence of osteomyelitis, gangrene, infection, ischemia, and neuropathy, but it does not include ulcer size, so this grading system is not used in isolation; however, it is predictive of outcomes, with grades 3 to 5 indicating marked compromise.

123. A: An older adult with a urinary infection may exhibit confusion rather than the more typical symptoms of burning and frequency experienced by younger adults, so urinary tract infection should be suspected in an older adult who has sudden onset of confusion or sudden worsening of

preexisting dementia. Confusion is more likely to occur with severe infections that have spread to the kidneys. The confusion associated with urinary tract infection usually clears rapidly once the infection is treated.

124. C: The statement by an AGACNP that demonstrates a good understanding of peer review is: "Peer review is a good learning experience for me and the person I'm reviewing." The point of peer review is that the reviews are done by peers, those of the same rank, and not supervisors and never anonymously. The reviewer and the reviewee should discuss the review with the reviewer prompting the reviewee to seek solutions to any problems that may have been identified.

125. B: If the AGACNP finds a patient with post-traumatic stress disorder (PTSD) and flashbacks cowering in the corner of the room in a state of panic, the best approach is to say, "I know you are afraid, but you are safe here." The AGACNP should acknowledge the patient's fears while trying to use grounding techniques to remind the patient that he is safe but should not attempt to reach out to the patient or touch the patient without first asking for permission because this may trigger a violent response.

126. D: If an insurer, such as Blue Cross/Blue Shield, denies a claim, an internal appeal (carried out by the insurance company) must be submitted within 180 days of the denial. The insurance company must complete the appeals process and render a decision within 30 days for future services and 60 days for services already received. If the insurer continues to deny the claim, the claimant has 60 days after notification of the denial to request an external review carried out by a third party.

127. B: The Mini-Cog test requires the person to remember and later repeat the names of three common objects and to draw the face of a clock with all 12 numbers and two hands indicating a specified time. The Mini-Mental State Examination (MMSE) requires a number of tasks, including counting backward from 100 by 7s, providing the current location, repeating phrases, following directions, and copying a picture of interlocking shapes. Instrumental Activities of Daily Living (IADLs) measure eight activities necessary for adults to function independently (including shopping, food preparation, telephone use, and managing finances). The Confusion Assessment Method is used to assess development of delirium, not dementia.

128. C: Transient ischemia attacks (TIAs) are usually diagnosed with carotid angiography to show intracranial and cervical circulation. Digital subtraction angiography defines the degree of carotid obstruction and shows patterns of cerebral blood flow. Symptoms of TIA typically persist for a few seconds or minutes but are always <24 hours. TIAs may indicate an impending stroke. Strokes are diagnosed initially with noncontrast computed tomography (CT) to determine if the stroke is hemorrhagic or ischemic. Other tests for stroke may include magnetic resonance imaging (MRI), transcranial Doppler flow studies, xenon-enhanced CT scanning, single-photon emission computed tomography (SPECT), and transthoracic/transesophageal echocardiography.

129. A: Barriers to systems thinking include a reliance on past experience. New directions require new solutions, so being mired in the past or relying solely on past experience can prevent progress. Systems thinking is having the background knowledge and practical tools to manage environmental and system resources, within and outside of the healthcare system, in order to solve problems for the patient/family and meet their needs. Other barriers include feelings of victimization, autocratic views, identification with role rather than purpose, failure to adapt, and weak consensus.

130. A: Although all of these elements are important, best practices identified through literature review should carry the most weight when developing evidence-based guidelines. Preferences are

often based on subjective rather than objective observations and may relate to familiarity and ease of use. Cost-effectiveness is always an issue and must be considered, but it should not be the primary concern. In some cases, spending more to prevent a problem initially may save money in terms of morbidity and extended medical care in the long-term.

131. B: If a 38-year-old female patient has had recurrent struvite (magnesium ammonium phosphate) urinary stones, the most appropriate treatment regimen includes antibiotics and acetohydroxamic acid. Struvite stones are formed as a result of a urinary tract infection, usually *Proteus* organisms, and occur three to four times more frequently in females than males. The antibiotic is used to destroy the bacteria, and the acetohydroxamic acid retards development of struvite stones in the presence of bacteria. Surgical removal of stones may be necessary.

132. D: The most important factor in cost management is eliminating duplication of services and care fragmentation. The AGACNP may also manage costs by conducting cost comparisons when obtaining supplies and equipment, but the least expensive option is not always the best, so quality is also a consideration. The AGACNP may exercise creativity and ingenuity in providing services in a cost-effective manner and may need to actively obtain data in order to show cost-effectiveness and influence coverage by the individual's insurance carrier.

133. C: The abbreviation of U for units is on the "Do Not Use" list. Other prohibited abbreviations/symbols include IU; QD; QOD; MS, MSO, and MgSO4 for morphine or magnesium sulfate; trailing zeros (4.0 mg) and lack of a leading zero (0.4 mg). Additional abbreviations/symbols are allowed but are under consideration for future prohibition. These include <, >, @, cc, µg, and abbreviations of drug names (such as TCN for tetracycline). Using the correct word or term is always better than using an abbreviation, which may be misunderstood, especially if writing is not clear.

134. B: These symptoms are consistent with hyperthyroidism, which poses a risk of adverse cardiac events, so the patient should be placed on a beta-blocker, such as Lopressor, for stabilization until further assessment by an endocrinologist. If patients are unable to take beta-blockers, they may be prescribed calcium channel blockers, although they may be less effective. Synthroid is used for hypothyroidism. Methimazole and propylthiouracil are both antithyroid medications, usually the treatment of choice because of risks associated with surgery, although thyroidectomy may be done in some cases.

135. D:

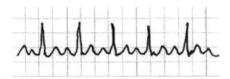

Atrial flutter (AF) occurs when the atrial rate is faster (usually 250–400 beats per minute) than the AV node conduction rate so that not all of the beats are conducted into the ventricles (ventricular rate 75–150), effectively being blocked at the AV node, preventing ventricular fibrillation, although some extra ventricular impulses may go through. AF is caused by the same conditions that cause atrial fibrillation: coronary artery disease, valvular disease, pulmonary disease, heavy alcohol ingestion, and cardiac surgery. Treatment includes the following:

Cardioversion if condition is unstable.

Medications to slow the ventricular rate and conduction through the AV node: Cardizem, Calan.

- 54 -

Medications to convert to sinus rhythm: Corvert, Cardioquin, Norpace, Cordarone.

136. A: Immobility is one of the most common nondisease causes of illness. Immobility, whether enforced by disability or chosen, may result in extended bedrest or sitting in a chair (such as those who watch TV hour after hour). Immobility can lead to deep vein thrombosis, pneumonia, constipation, urinary tract infection, pressure sores, kidney stones, muscle weakness, exercise intolerance, obesity, and depression. Prolonged bedrest has especially profound negative effects on the body.

137. A: With this presentation, the most likely diagnosis is scabies, which is caused by the Sarcoptes scabiei mite. A magnifying glass and penlight aimed at an oblique angle is used to help identify burrows. Scabies is highly contagious and nursing personnel in contact with the patient may become infected. Treatment is with a scabicide and oral antihistamine to control pruritis.

138. C: To evaluate cranial nerve X (vagus), ask the patient to swallow and speak, observing for difficulty in swallowing or hoarseness, and stimulate the back of the tongue or pharynx to elicit the gag reflex. Other examinations include:

- Cranial nerve IX (glossopharyngeal): Observe the patient swallowing, and place sugar or salt at the back third of his or her tongue to determine if the patient can differentiate between them.
- Cranial nerve XI (spinal accessory): Place your hands on the patient's shoulders and ask him or her to shrug against resistance.
- Cranial nerve XII (hypoglossal): Ask the patient to protrude the tongue and move it from side to side against a tongue depressor.

139. D: The bacterial infection that is most often associated with the development of Guillain-Barré syndrome (GBS) is *Campylobacter jejuni.* About 75% of patients with GBS have a preceding bacterial or viral infection, which is believed to trigger an autoimmune response. *C. jejuni* infection is most often acquired through eating undercooked meat, unpasteurized milk, and home-canned foods. Viral infections such as cytomegalovirus, human immunodeficiency virus (HIV), and Epstein-Barr virus may also trigger GBS.

140. C: Justice is the ethical principle that relates to the distribution of the limited resources of healthcare benefits to the members of society. These resources must be distributed fairly. This issue may arise if there is only one bed left and two sick patients. Justice comes into play in deciding which patient should stay and which should be transported or otherwise cared for. The decision should be made according to what is best or most just for the patients and not influenced by personal bias.

141. C: For Medicare reimbursement, if a physician received $192 for a procedure (out of a $240 charge), the AGACNP would receive 85% of the amount the physician received if billing for the same procedure. Medicare reimburses 80% (of usual and customary charges), and the patient or a secondary insurance is responsible for 20%. Thus, if the physician billed $240 and received 80% ($192) from Medicare, the nurse would bill 85% of $192 and would receive $163.20.

142. B: If a patient with a history alcoholism and cirrhosis has signs of portal hypertension, including abdominal ascites, the patient should be assessed for esophageal and gastric varices because she is at risk for GI bleeding because the varices may spontaneously rupture. The patient may also show evidence of encephalopathy and an impaired immune system (thrombocytopenia [secondary to alcoholic bone marrow suppression] and leukopenia [secondary to enlarged spleen]).

Noninvasive imaging, such as Doppler ultrasound, is used to assess liver size and to establish the patency of portal, splenic, and hepatic veins.

143. D: The AGACNP should recommend the pneumococcal vaccination (PCV13) (Prevnar13) to adults 65 and older. One year after receiving PCV13, the patient should receive vaccination with pneumococcal polysaccharide vaccine (PPSV23) (Pneumovax23). Contraindications to the vaccinations include allergy to any components. These vaccinations prevent many types of pneumococcal diseases, including pneumonia, ear infections, sinus infections, meningitis, and bacteremia.

144. A: Because of high risk, the AGACNP should screen bariatric patients for depression and eating disorders. Bariatric patients are especially susceptible to depression and may eat excessively because of being depressed and/or may become depressed because of the inability to control weight or the response of others to obesity. Additionally, patients are especially at risk for bulimia, often gorging and purging in cycles.

145. B: Class II.

Hemorrhagic shock classification		
Class	Blood loss	Signs and symptoms
I	≤15% (up to 750 mL)	Mild tachycardia (90–100 bpm), localized swelling, and frank bleeding. BP normal. Respirations 14–20. Urine: >30 mL/hr. Patient is slightly anxious.
II	15 to 25% (750–1500 mL)	Tachycardia (>100), prolonged capillary refill and increased diastolic BP. Respirations 20–30. Urine 20–30 mL/hr. Patient is mildly anxious.
III	25 to 50% (1500–2000 mL)	Above signs (any), tachycardia (>120) as well as hypotension, confusion, decreased urinary output, and acidosis. Respirations 30–40. Urine: 5–15 mL/hr. Patient is anxious and confused.
IV	>50% (>200 mL)	Tachycardia (>140), hypotension and acidosis unresponsive to resuscitation. Respirations >35. Urine: Scant. Patient is confused and lethargic.

146. C: If a patient is hospitalized with an acute myocardial infarction with ST segment elevation, a 50% reduction in mortality rates occurs if the patient is treated with thrombolytic therapy within 3 hours. Thrombolytic agents include streptokinase, tenecteplase, reteplase, and alteplase, although streptokinase is now rarely used because it is less effective than the other drugs. Following thrombolysis, the patient is continued on acetylsalicylic acid (ASA) therapy indefinitely and heparin for the first few days.

147. A: If a patient presents in the emergency department after falling from a horse and being kicked in the left side and has a fractured left lower rib and is exhibiting elevation of the left hemidiaphragm, left lower lobe atelectasis, and pleural effusion as well as tachycardia, hypotension, left flank pain, and positive Kehr's sign (pain referred to left shoulder), the AGACNP should recognize these signs and symptoms as indications of a ruptured spleen. Immediate surgical exploration may be needed to prevent the patient from bleeding out.

148. D: Respiratory alkalosis almost always results from hyperventilation. Hyperventilation decreases the $PaCO_2$ level in the blood as well as the carbonic acid level. This in turn results in increased pH and alkalosis. Laboratory findings include:

Increased serum pH >7.45.

Decreased $PaCO_2$ <38 mm Hg.

HCO_3 is normal if uncompensated and decreased if compensated.

Urine pH >6 if compensated.

Electrolytes: Hypokalemia and hypocalcemia.

Signs and symptoms of respiratory alkalosis include confusion, numbness, hyperreflexia, tetany, tachycardia, dysrhythmias, nausea, vomiting, and obvious hyperventilation.

149. A: Nicotine (smoking) is a precipitating factor for angina that results in sympathetic nervous system stimulation and release of catecholamines, which increase the heart rate and cause vasoconstriction. Additionally, the oxygen that is available to the heart is decreased because of increased carbon monoxide levels. Carbon monoxide displaces oxygen on the hemoglobin. Other precipitating factors may include exertion, temperature extremes, emotional changes, stimulant drugs, and sexual activity.

150. A: An exercise electrocardiogram (ECG) (stress test) is contraindicated for a patient who has chest pain at rest or on minimal exertion. Patients should avoid taking sildenafil citrate (Viagra) for at least 24 hours prior to the test because they may need nitroglycerin if chest pain occurs during the test and the combination of drugs may cause precipitous hypotension. Patients unable to take the exercise ECG may have a chemical stress test with an IV agent, such as dobutamine, adenosine, or dipyridamole.

151. B: If a male patient with a history of antisocial personality asks the female AGACNP if she spent the weekend with her boyfriend, the most appropriate response is "It's not appropriate to ask the nursing staff personal questions." The AGACNP must avoid overreacting or threatening but must identify acceptable behavior and limits because patients with antisocial personality disorder tend to be very manipulative.

152. D: The most effective treatment of trigeminal neuralgia is generally carbamazepine or oxcarbazepine (although the latter drug is not FDA approved for this condition). If carbamazepine is not tolerated, then phenytoin, baclofen, lamotrigine, or gabapentin may be tried. Trigeminal neuralgia is characterized by severe stabbing facial pains aggravated by touch, movement, air movement, and eating. Patients may benefit from gamma radiosurgery to the trigeminal root or surgical decompression with separation of an anomalous vein from the nerve.

153. C: Although magnetic resonance imaging (MRI) is more accurate in diagnosing breast cancer, MRI is also more expensive, so it is usually reserved for those who have greater than a 20% risk of lifetime development of breast cancer (such as those with a BRCA mutation or other high-risk mutations). The MRI is able to identify occult lesions smaller than those the mammogram identifies; however, it cannot distinguish between benign and malignant lesions, so an ultrasound may be done after an MRI to help distinguish benign from malignant masses.

154. A: If a 27-year-ld male with lower back pain and stiffness that improve with activity but are progressing upward is diagnosed with ankylosing spondylitis, the initial treatment regimen includes a nonsteroidal anti-inflammatory drug (NSAID). Patients may react differently to different NSAIDs, so empiric trials may be necessary. The onset of ankylosing spondylitis is gradual, usually beginning with back pain and stiffness on awakening in the morning. Over time, chest expansion may become limited. About 50% develop arthritis in peripheral joints as well.

155. D: The most common cause of medical error is communication problems, resulting in the widest range of errors in all levels of patient care. Communication problems often occur at hand-off when important information is omitted, so using a standardized format may help to reduce error. Other causes of medical error include inadequate flow of information (such as timely lab reports), lack of knowledge or failure to follow procedures, failure to properly identify the patient, inadequate training, staffing problems, equipment failure, and inadequate procedures and policies.

156. B: The drug of choice for mild to moderate *Clostridium difficile* infection is metronidazole (500 mg three times a day [TID] × 10 days). However, if the infection is severe and/or life threatening, then metronidazole should not be used, but treatment may include vancomycin (125 mg to 500 mg once a day [QID] × 10 days) or fidaxomicin (200 mg two times a day [BID] × 10 days). For those with recurrent infection, a fecal transplant is recommended. The best overall preventive to *Clostridium difficile* infections is to avoid overuse of broad-spectrum antibiotics.

157. A: When the AGACNP is educating a patient with a familial history of rheumatoid arthritis (RA), the patient should be advised to stop smoking because smoking has been linked to the development of RA as well as the severity of the disease. Even after smoking cessation, the increased risk of developing the disease remains for about 20 years. Researchers estimate that about 50% of the risk of developing RA is genetic but that smoking accounts for about 20% of overall cases.

158. C: When faced with a problem, such as a patient complaining of postoperative pain, the easiest approach is solution focused. These actions would include administering pain mediation, instructing the patient in visualization and relaxation, and ordering a stronger pain medication. A cause-focused solution, on the other hand, attempts to identify the cause of the problem before deciding on a solution. This may include examining a wound for signs of infection or complications (dressing too tight), checking vital signs and laboratory reports, and talking to and observing the patient.

159. D: In response to decreased renal perfusion or decreased sodium intake, the kidneys secrete renin into the circulatory system. Renin then converts angiotensinogen (produced by the liver) into angiotensin I. A pulmonary enzyme (angiotensin-converting enzyme) then further converts the angiotensin I to angiotensin II, which stimulates the production and release of aldosterone by the adrenal glands. Aldosterone functions to conserve sodium and increase excretion of potassium in order to increase blood pressure by increasing the volume of extracellular fluid.

160. B: If a coworker claims to have disposed of narcotics without a witness and asks the AGACNP to sign after the fact, the most appropriate action is to refuse to sign because of complicity. This is a common method of diversion and should be reported to a supervisor. Disposal should be witnessed by at least two healthcare providers who are licensed to dispense drugs. Disposal (such as when only 1 mL of a 2 mL vial is used) should be done immediately.

161. A: Total loss of respiratory muscle function occurs with spinal cord injuries above C4. The diaphragm is innervated by the phrenic nerve (C3 to C5), so injury above this level requires

immediate intubation and ventilation. Even with injuries below C4, the intercostal muscles may be paralyzed, resulting in hypoventilation. If the abdominal muscles are paralyzed, then the patient may be unable to cough or clear the airway. Those with injuries at C5 or higher usually have a tracheostomy performed to facilitate mechanical ventilation.

162. C: The lifestyle change that the AGACNP should recommend to a patient with obstructive sleep apnea is to stop smoking. Smokers have three times the risk of developing obstructive sleep apnea than nonsmokers, and the inflammation resulting from smoking can worsen the disorder. The patient should be referred to a smoking cessation program. Nicotine replacement products (gum, patches) may cause the patient difficulty with getting and staying asleep, so they should be prescribed with care.

163. D: If a 40-year-old patient is diagnosed with latent autoimmune diabetes in adults (LADA) (aka "slow diabetes" or "diabetes 1.5"), the duration of time from onset of symptoms to insulin dependence is usually about 2 to 4 years (compared to 6 months for diabetes mellitus, type 1). Destruction of the beta cells that secrete insulin occurs but at a slower rate with destruction faster in younger patients than older ones. The usual age of onset is 30 to 50 years.

164. B: Alginate dressings (AlgiSite, Hydrofiber) come in wafers, ropes, and fibers. They are made from brown seaweed, which is very absorbent, so they absorb large amounts of exudate and then form a hydrophilic gel that fills and conforms to the shape of the wound. Alginate dressings may be used with full-thickness wounds, infected wounds, and wounds with undermining and tunneling. When applying alginates, they should be packed loosely into the wound to allow them room to swell. Alginates are covered with secondary dressings.

165. A: If a patient has acute pancreatitis and has an order for a histamine-2 receptor antagonist (ranitidine), the purpose of this drug is to decrease production of hydrochloric acid (HCL). HCL is produced in the stomach to digest food, especially fats, and it enters the small intestine as part of chyme. HCL stimulates the pancreas to produce pancreatic enzymes, but during acute pancreatitis, especially with obstruction, the enzymes may further damage the pancreas.

166. D: If a 16-year-old patient experienced a concussion when he was tackled by another player while playing football and lost consciousness for about 20 seconds and has some persistent confusion, the concussion would be classified as grade 3.

Concussion grading system (American Academy of Neurology)	
Grade 1	Transient confusion without loss of consciousness with symptoms resolving in <15 minutes.
Grade 2	Transient confusion without loss of consciousness with symptoms resolving in >15 minutes.
Grade 3	Any loss of consciousness of any duration, regardless of extent of confusion.

167. C: Phase III, Proliferation.

Wound healing process	
Phase I: Hemostasis	Within minutes: Platelets seal vessels, vasoconstriction occurs, and thrombin stimulates clotting and forms a fibrin mesh.
Phase II: Inflammation	Day 1 to days 4–6: This period is characterized by erythema, edema, and pain. Phagocytosis begins to clean the wound.
Phase III: Proliferation	Days 5 to 20: Fibroblasts produce collagen, granulation starts to form, epithelialization occurs, and a scar forms.
Phase IV: Maturation	Days 21+, remodeling phase: Fibroblasts leave the wound and collagen tightens, reducing scarring. The tissue gains tensile strength and the wound closes. Underlying tissue repairs itself over up to 18 months.

168. B: The class of compression stocking that is most appropriate for prevention of venous ulcers in patients at risk is class 2 (30 to 40 mm Hg) with about 35 mm Hg being ideal if patients are able to tolerate that amount of compression. The classes of compression stockings are listed as follows:

- Class 1: 20–30 mm Hg: Used for patients with varicose veins.
- Class 2: 30–40 mg: Used to prevent venous ulcers.
- Class 3: 40–50 mm Hg. Used for refractory venous ulcers and lymphedema.
- Class 4: 50–60 mm Hg: Used for lymphedema.

Compression stockings must be fitted and applied properly or they may do more harm than good.

169. A: If a 33-year-old patient developed hemorrhagic colitis after ingesting *Escherichia coli* (Shiga toxin-producing *E. coli* [STEC] O157:H7) in contaminated produced, the treatment that is indicated is supportive care only, including IV fluids and electrolytes. Antibiotics are not advised because they do not improve the course of the disease, they do increase the risk of renal complications, and they may contribute to antibiotic resistance. Most people recover within 12 days without treatment; however, about 5% go on to develop hemolytic uremic syndrome, primarily young children and older adults.

170. D: If a patient is admitted with possible Guillain-Barré syndrome (GBS) because of respiratory distress and weakness, the AGACNP recognizes that the weakness that is characteristic of GBS is ascending and symmetrical. Patients often have pain in the back and legs and burning, tingling, and shock-like sensations in the lower legs. About 40% of those with GBS develop respiratory impairment and/or failure. Symptoms usually peak after about 3 weeks, although many have prolonged residual weakness.

171. C: If a patient reports the sudden appearance of a large number of cherry angiomas on her abdomen, the AGACNP should recognize that this may be a sign of internal malignancy and order further testing. Cherry angiomas are common lesions that can be found anywhere on the body and are usually benign. They are vascular lesions, so they can bleed freely if traumatized.

172. A: If a 72-year-old stroke patient has daily physical therapy that includes assisted walking on a treadmill, and a large mirror is placed in front of the treadmill, the purpose of the mirror is to

- 60 -

provide visual feedback. The feedback helps the patient to recognize positioning because this sense is often impaired in stroke patients. There is some belief that observing the unaffected body part moving may help to stimulate movement on the affected side.

173. D: If the AGACNP prescribes disulfiram to a patient for alcohol dependence, the patient should be advised that after stopping the medication, a disulfiram-alcohol reaction can occur for up to 2 weeks. The first dose should be taken at least 12 hours after the last drink. Because the drug inhibits metabolism of alcohol, drinking will result in flushing, nausea, vomiting, and tachycardia.

174. B: If a patient with obsessive-compulsive disorder is hospitalized with a myocardial infarction (MI) and uses ritualized number patterns of behavior, such as emptying water out of a glass four times before drinking from the glass, the AGACNP recognizes that the primary rationale for this behavior is to reduce anxiety. Staff members should be advised not to interfere with ritualized behavior unless it poses a risk to the patient or others.

175. C: When treating a patient for increased intracranial pressure (ICP), the goal should be to maintain the ICP within the normal range and the cerebral perfusion pressure (CPP) at greater than 60 mm Hg. If the blood pressure falls, especially with aggressive treatment of increased ICP, the CPP will decrease, so maintaining the blood pressure and even tolerating some hypertension is critical because the body may attempt to maintain the CPP by increasing the blood pressure.

176. A: If, when describing chest pain, the patient runs the fingers of both hands up and down either side of the sternum, the most likely origin of the pain is the gastrointestinal (GI) system (such as the esophagus). This is a fairly typical description of heartburn or indigestion with reflux. The pain may increase when the patient is in the supine position. Heartburn may be described further as a "burning" pain. The pain may be relieved with antacids.

177. C: When educating a patient with coronary artery disease about managing anginal episodes, the AGACNP advises the patient to take nitroglycerin one time and then call 9-1-1 prior to the second dose if the pain persists. This allows the patient to get faster attention if he or she is having a heart attack. The previous recommendations (take the pills three times 5 minutes apart before calling 9-1-1) delayed treatment, resulting in higher morbidity/mortality.

178. B: The risk factor that places a female at highest risk for myocardial infarction is having diabetes mellitus. Other first-tier risk factors include coronary heart disease, cerebrovascular disease, peripheral arterial disease, abdominal aortic aneurysm, and chronic or end-stage renal disease. Smoking, obesity, and hypertension as well as poor diet, inactivity, dyslipidemia, and metabolic syndrome are second-tier risk factors.

179. D: If a patient involved in a frontal-impact motor vehicle accident arrives at the emergency department with a markedly widened mediastinum, left hemothorax, and transient hypotension, based on these findings, the AGACNP should alert the staff that the patient likely has aortic rupture. Aortic rupture usually occurs from blunt trauma to the chest. This is an emergent situation that requires immediate surgical repair because death often occurs within 30 minutes.

180. D: If a certified nursing assistant (CNA) tells the AGACNP that when doing range-of-motion (ROM) exercises on a bedridden patient, the CNA meets resistance when trying to completely extend the right elbow, the AGACNP should advise the CNA to extend the arm only to the point of resistance. The AGACNP should also evaluate the arm to determine the cause of the limitation and to consider whether a referral to a physical therapist is indicated.

181. A: When discussing safety issues with team members, the AGACNP reminds the team that the best way to prevent falls is to use strategies appropriate for each patient. A patient with dementia, for example, may need a movement alarm, whereas a more alert patient may need a light on in the bathroom at night. In all cases, the environment should be kept clear of obstructions and patients should be monitored frequently.

182. B: If a patient hospitalized with an ischemic stroke develops a hypertensive emergency, the recommended drug treatment includes nicardipine, clevidipine, or labetalol. Drugs that are contraindicated include nitroprusside, methyldopa, clonidine, and nitroglycerin. Nitroprusside may decrease cerebral blood flow. Clonidine may increase sedation. Nitroglycerin may result in hypotension and decreased cerebral blood flow. Immediate treatment is essential to prevent further cerebrovascular injury, but hypotension must be avoided, so the BP reduction must be carefully monitored.

183. D: Green.

Color codes for emergency/disaster situations	
Red (priority)	Unconscious, altered mental status, chest pain, chest wounds, severe burns, hemorrhage, amputation (above knee or above elbow), abnormal pulse, open abdominal wounds, spinal cord injuries.
Yellow (serious)	Deep lacerations, open fractures, multiple fractures, digit amputations, closed-head injuries but alert, abdominal injuries but stable vital signs.
Green (minor)	Abrasions, contusions, minor lacerations, sprains, and other mild injuries. No injuries.
Black (dead/dying)	Injuries appear inconsistent with life, or the patient is already deceased.

184. A: If a patient has had a thumb reattached but the thumb is congested because only the arteries and not the veins were reattached, leech therapy may be used to drain the congested blood. After the leech is attached, the patient should be monitored continuously during the 15–20 minutes of treatment to make sure that it does not wander or detach. During treatment, the leech usually drains 5 to 15 mL of blood, but the attachment site continues to drain for hours, resulting in blood loss of 50 to 150 mL.

185. C: If, during a patient's physical examination, the AGACNP asks the patient to frown, smile, close eyes tightly against resistance, show teeth, lift eyebrows, and puff out the cheeks, the cranial nerve that the AGACNP is assessing is cranial nerve VII, the facial nerve. Flattening of the nasolabial fold, lower eyelid sagging, unilateral drooping of the face, and air leaking from one side of the cheek with pressure indicate muscle weakness. Impaired movement and asymmetry may result from either central nervous system (CNS) or peripheral nervous system (PNS) lesions.

186. B: With chronic mitral regurgitation, the heart chamber that enlarges first is the left atrium, which may become greatly enlarged. The left ventricle also becomes enlarged over time because of volume overload, and this can lead to atrial fibrillation, left ventricular failure, and reduced cardiac output. Mitral regurgitation can be identified by a pansystolic murmur, maximal at the apex and radiating to the axilla. A prominent third heart sound results from increased volume returning to the left ventricle.

187. C: Both male and female hormones are normally metabolized by the liver. If a 64-year-old male patient with cirrhosis of the liver has developed gynecomastia, the primary reason is an impaired ability to metabolize estrogen, so the estrogen level increases. The increased estrogen stimulates growth of the breast tissue. The patient may also experience decreased axillary and pubic hair, testicular atrophy, and impaired libido or impotence. Females have increased male hormones resulting in amenorrhea for younger women and vaginal bleeding for older women as well as hypernatremia, water retention, and hypokalemia.

188. D: If a patient who has had a pacemaker implanted for bradycardia is to be discharged asks the AGACNP about driving, the patient should be advised to avoid driving for 1 month. This gives the tissue time to heal around the pacemaker and gives enough time to ensure that the pacemaker is functioning properly and that the patient has no residual problems, such as dizziness, that might make driving unsafe.

189. A: If an abdominal CT has indicated that a patient has a large tumor low in the descending colon, the signs and symptoms that are characteristic include pain, change in bowel habits, and bright-red blood in the stool. In some cases, complete bowel obstruction may occur. With a tumor in this site, the patient will likely have a colostomy placed in the descending colon, meaning that the stool will be formed and evacuation is controlled with regular irrigations.

190. C: When initiating digoxin therapy for heart failure, the blood level of the drug should be measured within 1 to 2 weeks. The test should be done at least 6 hours after the last administered dose. The level should be maintained between 0.7 ng/mL and 1.2 ng/mL. Higher rates may result in increased risk of arrhythmias and increased mortality rates. Toxicity is usually evident with levels of 1.8 or higher. The therapeutic dose to toxic dose ratio is quite narrow, so patients should be apprised of signs of digitalis toxicity (anorexia, nausea, headache, blurred yellowing vision, and disorientation).

191. B: If a 17-year-old male patient who is tall with abnormally long arms, legs, and fingers and has a chest abnormality (pectus excavatum) is diagnosed with Marfan syndrome, the annual surveillance that is indicated is an eye exam and echocardiogram. Marfan syndrome affects the ocular system, so the patient must have regular eye exams to correct visual acuity. An echocardiogram is critical to assess the aorta because of the risk of aortic regurgitation or dissection. About 85% of patients have mitral valve prolapse.

192. A: If a 58-year-old patient was admitted with severe acute pancreatitis, the finding 24 hours after admission and beginning of treatment indicating a worsening prognosis is a drop in the hematocrit value of greater than 10%. Other signs of worsening condition include the following:

- Blood urea nitrogen (BUN) increase greater than 5 mg/dL.
- Arterial PO_2 of less than 60 mm Hg.
- Serum calcium of less than 8 mg/dL.
- Base deficit of greater than 4 mEq/L.
- Estimated fluid sequestration of greater than 6L.

193. D: If a 26-year-old patient has symptoms of chronic endometriosis (growth of endometrial tissue outside of the uterus, especially in the ovaries and dependent parts of pelvis) with pelvic pain, dysmenorrhea, and dyspareunia, the imaging modality of choice for diagnosis is transvaginal ultrasonography, although imaging has limited value. A definitive diagnosis is made through histology of surgically excised lesions. Treatment usually includes low-dose combined

contraceptives (oral, patches, vaginal rings). Endometriosis is associated with infertility, especially with ovarian involvement.

194. C: If a recent outbreak of *Giardia* infection from an infected public pool has brought many patients to the emergency room, the public should be advised that, after ingestion of cysts, symptoms usually begin within 1 to 2 weeks. About 15% are asymptomatic, but about 50% have GI upset and diarrhea, abdominal pain, flatulence, fatty stools, cramping, nausea, vomiting and weight loss (typically about 15 pounds in an adult). Symptoms usually persist for 1 to 3 weeks, and some may develop chronic disease. The treatment of choice is metronidazole 250 mg TID for 5 to 7 days.

195. B: If, when conducting a physical examination of a 50-year-old patient, the AGACNP notes that the patient has spoon-shaped nails, this most commonly indicates an iron deficiency anemia. Pitted nails are an indication of psoriasis. Patient with chronic hypoxia may have clubbing of the nails and a straightening of the angle between the nail and the base to 180° or greater. Trauma to the nail may result in ridges, hypertrophy, or other changes.

196. A: If a patient with cervical cancer is treated with high-dose radiation (HDR) brachytherapy (intracavity), the other interventions that are necessary during the 72 hours of treatment include bedrest, low-residue diet, antidiarrheal medication, and indwelling urinary catheter. Any straining, such as to urinate or defecate, or the pressure of a full bladder may dislodge the implant. The patient is placed in a specially prepared room with notices to warn staff of the necessary precautions. All staff should wear a dosimeter while in the room and stay for only short periods.

197. D: <u>Macular</u> lesions are <1 cm, flat, and nonpalpable with a circumscribed border. Macules >1 cm are <u>patches</u>. <u>Papular</u> lesions are <0.5 cm in diameter, elevated, palpable with a solid mass and circumscribed border. If >0.5 cm, they are <u>plaques</u>. <u>Nodular</u> lesions are elevated and palpable with a solid mass that extend deeper into the tissue than papules and are 0.5 to 2 cm in diameter with circumscribed borders. If >1 to 2 cm and without clearly defined borders, they are <u>tumors</u>. <u>Vesicular</u> lesions are <0.5 cm, elevated, circumscribed, palpable, and filled with fluid. If they are > 0.5 cm, they are <u>bullae</u>.

198. C: If a patient's nursing diagnosis is "Ineffective airway clearance associated with edema and the effects of smoke inhalation," the goal should be to maintain a patent airway and adequate airway clearance. As much as possible, the goal should reflect the issues outlined in the nursing diagnosis as well as the expected outcomes. The interventions should be those that help to achieve the stated goals, such as proper positioning, use of an incentive spirometer, providing humidified oxygen, and encouraging the patient to deep-breathe and cough.

199. B: The most common cause of visual loss for people older than age 60 in the United States is macular degeneration. The two types include the dry (nonneovascular) type, in which the outer layers of the retina deteriorate creating drusen, which may cause gradual blurring of vision. The wet (neovascular) type of macular degeneration) occurs when abnormal blood vessels proliferate under the retina, resulting in vision distortions (wavy lines, crooked letters). Dry macular degeneration is treated with macronutrients, and wet macular degeneration is treated with antiangiogenic therapy.

200. C: Fragile X is an X-linked recessive genetic disorder that affects males, but females may inherit a carrier state and may exhibit some symptoms (although they are milder than in males). Up to 25% of females who are carriers and carry the FMR1 gene develop fragile X-associated primary ovarian insufficiency, which is characterized by subfertility, infertility, and early-onset menopause,

usually by age 40. The number and quality of ova may also be affected. Some women are able to get pregnant, but they are at risk of having a child with fragile X syndrome.

Practice Test #2

1. For patients with diabetes mellitus, the first indication of diabetic nephropathy is usually:

    a. increased creatinine.
    b. increased blood urea nitrogen (BUN).
    c. microalbuminuria.
    d. macroalbuminuria.

2. A 36-year-old male patient has acute sexually transmitted epididymitis. In addition to antibiotics during the acute phase of the disease, the treatment regimen should include:

    a. warm compresses.
    b. ice compresses.
    c. scrotal support.
    d. bed rest and scrotal elevation.

3. A patient with burns is placed on an air-fluidized bed to relieve pressure. It is especially important to carefully monitor this patient for:

    a. vital signs.
    b. fluid balance.
    c. temperature.
    d. pain level.

4. At what body mass index (BMI) are patients considered obese and should be counseled regarding diet, lifestyle choices, and weight loss goals?

    a. ≥ 30.
    b. ≥ 28.
    c. ≥ 26.
    d. ≥ 25.

5. A 68-year-old patient has been treated for renal disease but has exhibited a sudden change in her condition. The primary indications for renal replacement therapy (RRT) for acute renal failure are:

    a. hypovolemia, metabolic alkalosis, and hypokalemia.
    b. initial signs of oliguria.
    c. increasing levels of serum creatinine.
    d. fluid overload, metabolic acidosis, and hyperkalemia.

6. After removal of a chest tube, a 48-year-old patient complains of retrosternal and neck pain, is dyspneic, and has slight neck edema. Hamman's sign is positive (precordial systolic crepitus). The probable diagnosis is:

    a. pneumothorax.
    b. cardiac tamponade.
    c. pneumomediastinum.
    d. pneumopericardium.

7. Phase I of becoming bedridden (Zegelin, 2008) begins with:

    a. a fall.
    b. unstable gait/imbalance.
    c. prolonged prescribed bed rest and chair.
    d. prolonged continuous bed rest.

8. Which of the following antidysrhythmic drugs is most likely to result in bradycardia, hypotension, heart failure, PR prolongation, and/or constipation?

    a. Lidocaine.
    b. Ibutilide.
    c. Amiodarone.
    d. Diltiazem.

9. Which of the following best describes Kolb's model of experiential learning?

    a. Knowledge develops from experience interacting with cognition and perception.
    b. Knowledge and experience are equally important.
    c. Experience precedes knowledge in learning.
    d. Learning cannot be acquired without experience and perception.

10. If a patient reports that injuries resulted from domestic violence, when documenting the abuse in the patient's health record, the adult gerontology acute care nurse practitioner (AGACNP) should:

    a. summarize the patient's statements.
    b. indicate only that abuse occurred.
    c. use direct quotations to document the patient's statements.
    d. record no information but fill out an incident report.

11. A prevention strategy that encourages physicians, nurses, and other healthcare providers to discuss substance abuse with all adolescents is an example of:

    a. secondary prevention.
    b. universal primary prevention.
    c. indicated primary prevention.
    d. targeted primary prevention.

12. Because combining monoamine oxidase inhibitors (MAOIs) with some foods may cause adverse reactions (hypertension, headache, diaphoresis, cardiac abnormalities, intracerebral hemorrhage), patients taking MAOIs should be advised to avoid which of the following foods/beverages?

    a. Alcohol and grapefruit juice.
    b. Alcohol, products containing caffeine (tea, cola, chocolate coffee), and foods high in tyramine (organ meats, cured meats, cheese, raisins, avocados, and soy).
    c. Foods high in vitamin K (broccoli, spinach, Brussels sprouts, cauliflower, kale) and vitamin E supplements.
    d. Milk products and vitamins, vitamins and minerals containing iron, and caffeine.

13. Mike Brown has completed gender reassignment surgery (male-to-female) and is now legally Mikaela Brown. Mikaela states that she is still attracted to females and not males. Her sexual orientation should be most appropriately classified as:

    a. lesbian.
    b. heterosexual.
    c. homosexual.
    d. bisexual.

14. In conducting evidence-based research, which of the following types of studies represents one in which those with a condition (such as infection) are compared to those without the condition?

    a. Retrospective cohort study.
    b. Prospective cohort study.
    c. Case control study.
    d. Cross-sectional study.

15. When instituting suicide precautions, which patient is likely at highest risk?

    a. A 15-year-old girl who overdosed on aspirin and then told her best friend.
    b. A 50-year-old woman who overdosed on pills and alcohol while her family was present.
    c. A 26-year-old man who threatened to jump out of a second-story window.
    d. A 38-year-old man who shot himself in the chest while alone at home.

16. Fifteen hours after a patient was involved in an accident that resulted in a comminuted fracture of the femur, the patient exhibits increasing dyspnea and tachypnea as well as confusion, difficulty speaking, and a petechial rash in the mouth and upper body. The most likely cause of this triad of symptoms is:

    a. pulmonary embolism.
    b. fat embolism syndrome.
    c. pneumonia.
    d. stroke.

17. Two staff nurses in the acute care unit disagree about the best way to carry out their duties, resulting in ongoing conflict and refusal to work together. The first step in resolving this conflict is to:

    a. allow both individuals to present their side of the conflict without bias.
    b. encourage them to reach a compromise.
    c. tell them they are violating professional standards of conduct.
    d. make a decision about the matter.

18. During the initial assessment, a 75-year-old female states she has had one fall in the past 4 months but had no residual injury. What, if any, further testing is immediately indicated?

    a. No further testing.
    b. Gait, balance, and get-up-and-go.
    c. X-ray of the hips and spine.
    d. Bone mass density testing.

19. With severe heart failure, ventricular remodeling may occur with the ventricle walls thinning and enlarging, resulting in a larger ventricular capacity. This, in turn, results in:

    a. increased ejection fraction.
    b. increased cardiac output.
    c. decreased cardiac output.
    d. fluid retention and vasoconstriction.

20. Norovirus may remain viable on environmental surfaces, such as furniture, for up to:

    a. 24 hours.
    b. 48 hours.
    c. 12 days.
    d. 28 days.

21. Recommendations for the use of restraint and seclusion in pediatric patients limit the time adolescents 15 to 17 should be restrained and/or secluded to no longer than:

    a. one hour.
    b. two hours.
    c. four hours.
    d. six hours.

22. When administering platelets to a patient, the infusion should be done:

    a. as fast as possible.
    b. as slow as possible.
    c. over 1 to 2 hours.
    d. over 2 to 4 hours.

23. Which type of dementia is especially characterized by changes in personality and behavior and difficulty using and understanding language?

    a. Alzheimer's disease.
    b. Parkinson's dementia.
    c. Normal pressure hydrocephalus.
    d. Frontotemporal dementia.

24. A 62-year-old homeless man hospitalized for pneumonia is to be discharged but has no place to go and no income. Which of the following is of primary importance in preparing for discharge?

    a. Specific directions for medication or treatments, including side effects.
    b. Information sheets outlining signs for all risk factors.
    c. List of safe shelters and assistance in applying for welfare assistance or Social Security.
    d. Follow-up appointment dates, with physicians, labs, or other healthcare providers.

25. Drug absorption may be impaired in gerontology patients because of:

    a. decreased splanchnic blood flow.
    b. body water volume fluctuations.
    c. decreased renal blood flow.
    d. changed hepatic volume.

26. Which of the following findings on physical assessment are consistent with osteoarthritis?

    a. Spindle-shaped swelling of soft tissue of proximal interphalangeal joints.
    b. Ulnar deviation of fingers.
    c. Swan-neck deformity of fingers.
    d. Hard, nontender nodules on distal and proximal interphalangeal joints.

27. A patient has a percutaneous endoscopic gastrostomy (PEG) and has developed leakage about the tube. What initial intervention is indicated?

    a. Check the balloon to ensure adequate inflation.
    b. Stabilize the tube with the bumper and external stabilizer.
    c. Replace the tube.
    d. Apply a barrier ointment.

28. For which of the following is a positive Murphy's sign an aid in diagnosis?

    a. Differentiating cholecystitis from choledocholithiasis.
    b. Diagnosing cholecystitis in geriatric patients.
    c. Diagnosing pancreatitis.
    d. Differentiating ascending cholangitis from pancreatitis.

29. A 40-year-old patient with bipolar disease has been well controlled with lithium, but she comes to the emergency department with influenza that has caused 2 days of severe vomiting and diarrhea. In response to the bipolar disease, the AGACNP's priority should be to immediately:

    a. decrease the dose of lithium.
    b. increase the dose of lithium.
    c. discontinue the lithium.
    d. obtain a lithium level.

30. The Hamilton Anxiety Rating Scale (HAM-A) scores (0–4) phrases that describe:

    a. abnormalities.
    b. feelings and symptoms.
    c. desires.
    d. likes and dislikes.

31. When marking a nasoenteric tube for an adult patient prior to insertion for enteric feedings, what measurements are needed?

    a. Nose to earlobe, earlobe to xiphoid process.
    b. Nose to earlobe, earlobe to xiphoid process, plus 6 inches (15 cm).
    c. Nose to earlobe, earlobe to xiphoid process, plus 8 to 10 inches (20–25 cm).
    d. Nose to earlobe, earlobe to xiphoid process, plus 12 to 14 inches (30–38 cm).

32. A 46-year-old patient with stage 2 gastric cancer refuses all treatment because of religious convictions. Which of the following is the most appropriate action?

    a. Provide the patient with facts about the disease, treatments, and prognosis.
    b. Ask family members to intervene.
    c. Remind the patient that he will die without treatment.
    d. Refer him to a psychologist.

33. A 33-year-old female is hospitalized for treatment of acute pyelonephritis and has been receiving IV fluids and ampicillin plus aminoglycoside for the past 5 days, but the patient's temperature remains elevated and she is still in pain and nauseated. The patient should likely be evaluated for:

    a. perinephric abscess.
    b. pelvic inflammatory disease.
    c. allergic reaction to drugs.
    d. urinary tract obstruction.

34. A patient who suffered a stroke has persistent dysphagia and cough, and the AGACNP is concerned that the patient may aspirate. Which of the following referrals is the most appropriate?

    a. Physical therapist.
    b. Occupational therapist.
    c. Respiratory therapist.
    d. Speech pathologist.

35. The AGACNP is working on a unit that has been understaffed. One of the nurses on the unit states that his blood pressure has increased because he dreads coming to work and feels that the organization doesn't value nurses or care about patients and that nothing will change. The AGACNP should recognize that the nurse is most at risk for:

    a. workplace violence.
    b. burnout.
    c. accidental injury.
    d. negligent patient care.

36. A 73-year-old patient is in the hospital with hypothermia because his daughter, who manages his finances, forgot to pay the heating bill, so the heat was shut off during a cold spell. This is an example of:

    a. physical abuse.
    b. abandonment.
    c. neglect.
    d. emotional abuse.

37. If the AGACNP is promoting evidence-based practice and using the PICOT format to pose a clinical question, the AGACNP would first focus on:

    a. personal interests.
    b. philosophy of care.
    c. placement of resources.
    d. patient population.

38. A 70-year-old female with chronic obstructive pulmonary disease (COPD) has experienced an exacerbation after contracting an upper respiratory infection. The patient's oxygen saturation level on admission is 84%. Blood gases are as follows: pH, 7.29; $PaCO_2$, 52 mm Hg; PaO_2, 53 mm Hg; and HCO_3, 25 mEq/L. Based on these findings, the acid-base imbalance the patient is experiencing is:

    a. respiratory alkalosis.
    b. respiratory acidosis.
    c. metabolic alkalosis.
    d. metabolic acidosis.

39. The AGACNP has been asked to serve as a coach for nurses in the medical-surgical unit. The AGACNP's initial action should be to:

    a. complete a needs assessment.
    b. announce the role.
    c. prepare a plan of action.
    d. ask the supervisor for guidance.

40. A 27-year-old male patient has experienced increased thirst and frequency of urination, including nocturia. He has had an increased appetite but lost 4 pounds in the previous 2-week period. Laboratory tests show a glucose level of 526 mg/dL (29.2 mmol/L), urine positive for glucose and ketones, and an acidic blood pH of 7.22. The blood pH is the result of:

    a. a normal finding.
    b. increased urinary output.
    c. increased fluid intake.
    d. increased ketone levels in blood.

41. A 32-year-old female reports repeated episodes of palpitation 6 to 10 times daily. The patient has experienced increased irritability, insomnia, heat intolerance, and eye irritation. The patient has lost 5 pounds in the previous month but has an increased appetite. Vital signs are BP, 170/86; P, 114; R, 20. Temperature is 37.5°C (99.5°F), and the electrocardiogram (ECG) shows atrial fibrillation. Which of the following diagnostic tests are most indicated?

    a. Renal function tests.
    b. Cardiac enzymes.
    c. Thyroid function tests.
    d. Liver function tests.

42. According to Drug Enforcement Administration (DEA) regulations for schedule II drugs, what is the refill limitation without renewal by a healthcare practitioner?

    a. 0 refills.
    b. 2 refills.
    c. 5 refills.
    d. 12 refills.

43. Which of the following characteristics helps to distinguish an asthma attack from a chronic obstructive pulmonary disease (COPD) exacerbation?

    a. Asthma lacks a genetic component.
    b. Most asthma patients are smokers.
    c. Onset of asthma is usually younger than age 30.
    d. Asthma attacks respond less quickly to treatment.

44. A patient with a T-6 spinal cord injury is lying flat in bed but suddenly exhibits blurred vision, severe headache, piloerection with flushing above the lesion and pallor below, and markedly elevated BP of 280/160. The first action should be to:

    a. check bladder.
    b. check bowels.
    c. loosen clothes.
    d. elevate the head of the bed to 45°.

45. Which of the following teaching strategies is the most efficient approach for a group of eight patients regarding the need for lifestyle changes required to manage hypertension and heart disease?

a. Discussion.
b. Lecture-discussion.
c. Role playing.
d. Demonstration/Return demonstration.

46. The "talk and die" phenomenon in which a patient loses consciousness after a blow to the head and then recovers and appears to be fine before suddenly developing severe symptoms of brain injury is typical of:

a. epidural hemorrhage.
b. subdural hemorrhage.
c. intracerebral hemorrhage.
d. subarachnoid hemorrhage.

47. When conducting a history and physical exam of a patient with dyspnea, the AGACNP discovers that the patient has smoked two packs (40 cigarettes) daily for at least 15 years. How many pack-years does this represent?

a. 10.
b. 20.
c. 30.
d. 40.

48. If a nonverbal patient with dementia is frowning and grimacing on movement, crying out periodically, and lying rigid or in the fetal position, the AGACNP should recognize that the patient is likely:

a. hungry.
b. angry
c. frightened.
d. in pain.

49. A 60-year-old African-American patient presented with a body mass index (BMI) of 32 kg/m², hemoglobin A1C level of 7.1, fasting serum glucose of 152 mg/dL (8.4 mmol/L), triglyceride level of 168, and high-density lipoprotein (HDL) level of 24 mg/dL. The patient is diagnosed with insulin resistance and diabetes mellitus, type 2. Which of the following is usually the drug of choice to initiate therapy?

a. Sulfonylureas, such as glimepiride.
b. Biguanides, such as metformin.
c. Meglitinides, such as repaglinide.
d. Alpha-glucosidase inhibitors, such as acarbose.

50. Following lunch at a restaurant, a 72-year-old female experiences a sudden episode of loss of vision in the right eye. At the same time, the patient feels dizzy and weak, and her speech is slightly garbled, but the symptoms clear within 15 to 20 minutes. The most likely diagnosis is

a. transient ischemic episode (TIE).
b. stroke.
c. allergic reaction.
d. panic attack.

51. Which of the following methods of wound debridement generally should be avoided?

    a. sharp debridement.
    b. irrigation.
    c. wet-to-dry dressings.
    d. chemical debridement.

52. The medical-surgical unit has experienced an outbreak of *Clostridium difficile* infections involving 10 patients over a 2-week period. In order to reduce further transmission of the infection, the AGACNP is working with staff members and should concentrate efforts on:

    a. contact precautions/hand hygiene.
    b. antibiotic stewardship.
    c. testing patient stool specimens.
    d. limiting patient contacts.

53. A 16-year-old comes to the emergency department with a sore reddened and blistering area on his left lower leg. The patient states that he believes he was bitten by a spider, but didn't actually see the spider. What differential diagnosis should the AGACNP suspect?

    a. Lyme disease.
    b. Scabies.
    c. Shingles.
    d. *Staphylococcus aureus* infection.

54. A patient with heart failure has developed pulmonary edema and has an audible wheeze with rales and rhonchi present throughout the lung fields. The patient is quite anxious. The patient is initially treated with oxygen at 15 L per nonrebreather mask, furosemide 60 mg IV, as well as nitroglycerine and nitroprusside to increase peripheral vasodilation and morphine to reduce anxiety. The initial goal of therapy should be to maintain the PaO_2 at greater than:

    a. 40 mm Hg.
    b. 60 mm Hg.
    c. 70 mm Hg.
    d. 80 mm Hg.

55. If a patient is taking atorvastatin for dyslipidemia, which of the following medications may the AGACNP recommend for its additive effect to reduce the risk of cardiac mortality resulting from dyslipidemia?

    a. Bile acid sequestrant.
    b. Cholesterol absorption inhibitor.
    c. Fibrate.
    d. Microsomal transfer protein (MTP) inhibitor.

56. If a patient has suspected heart failure, which of the following tests should the AGACNP expect will show the severity of the heart failure?

    a. C-reactive protein (CRP).
    b. Homocysteine.
    c. Ischemia modified albumin (IMA).
    d. B-type natriuretic peptide (BNP).

57. If the AGACNP is using the beliefs, values, meanings, goals, and relationships (BVMGR) rubric for implementing spiritual care, these aspects apply to the:

    a. AGACNP.
    b. culture.
    c. patient.
    d. organization.

58. A patient with pulmonary arterial hypertension (World Health Organization disease type II [WHO II]) has started treatment with combination therapy that initially includes ambrisentan 5 mg (Letairis) and tadalafil 20 mg (Adcirca) as well as supplementary oxygen for exertion. When educating the patient about disease management, the AGACNP should tell the patient to be especially alert for signs of:

    a. unusual bleeding.
    b. peripheral edema.
    c. headache.
    d. dizziness.

59. If a patient with inflammatory bowel disease (IBD) has periodic bouts of severe diarrhea but is unsure of the cause, the AGACNP should advise the patient to:

    a. maintain a food diary.
    b. avoid all milk products.
    c. increase fat in diet.
    d. increase fiber in diet.

60. An alert 70-year-old female patient hospitalized with a vertebral fracture and no previous history of incontinence has started having both urinary and fecal leakage. The AGACNP's initial response is to examine the patient for:

    a. urinary infection.
    b. medication reaction.
    c. fecal impaction.
    d. psychological factors.

61. If a patient with latex allergy is inadvertently exposed to latex and develops severe anaphylaxis with difficulty breathing, the priority intervention is to establish an airway and administer:

    a. oxygen.
    b. epinephrine.
    c. corticosteroid.
    d. albuterol inhaler.

62. Absorption of nutrients from the small bowel is often impaired in older adults because of:

    a. age-related cellular mutations.
    b. decreased muscular contractility.
    c. narrowing and lengthening of villi.
    d. broadening and shortening of villi.

63. A 22-year-old patient is on a strict vegan diet. The patient is most at risk for which type of blood disorder?

    a. Vitamin B_{12} deficiency.
    b. Iron deficiency anemia.
    c. Folic acid deficiency.
    d. Autoimmune hemolytic anemia.

64. If the AGACNP needs to delegate a task to a licensed vocational or practical nurse (LVN/LPN) but is unsure how the nurse performs because the AGACNP has not worked with this LVN/LPN before, the best initial approach is to:

    a. assign the task and try to observe the LVN/LPN.
    b. ask the LVN/LPN how he or she would go about doing the task.
    c. ask the opinion of nurses who have worked with the LVN/LPN before.
    d. outline specific steps to carrying out the task.

65. The AGACNP should recommend the herpes zoster (shingles) vaccine for:

    a. all adults.
    b. adults 45 and older.
    c. adults 60 and older.
    d. adults 65 and older.

66. The AGACNP notes that one nursing team member often avoids taking care of older patients and sometimes makes disparaging remarks about the elderly. The most appropriate response is for the AGACNP to:

    a. advise the nurse that ageism is inappropriate.
    b. discuss attitudes toward aging with the nurse.
    c. file a complaint against the nurse.
    d. avoid assigning the nurse to older patients.

67. Acute kidney injury may occur with sepsis because of:

    a. nephrotoxins.
    b. autoimmune response.
    c. urinary tract obstruction.
    d. decreased renal perfusion.

68. A patient with fulminant hepatic failure is not a candidate for liver transplant and has signs of increasing intracranial pressure. The AGACNP advises member of the care team to:

    a. elevate the head of the bed to 30° and pad the side rails.
    b. apply restraints to the patient.
    c. elevate the head of the bed to 60°–90°.
    d. keep the patient heavily sedated.

69. At what blood alcohol level does a patient typically begin experiencing blackouts?

    a. 0.07 to 0.9 g/100 mL.
    b. 0.1 to 0.125 g/100 mL.
    c. 0.20 g/100 mL.
    d. 0.30 g/100 mL.

70. In order to optimize venous return and prevent pressure areas for a patient who is bedridden or has limited activity, as much as possible, the head of the patient's bed should be maintained at:

    a. ≤90°.
    b. ≤60°.
    c. ≤45°.
    d. ≤30°.

71. An 80-year-old patient with a history of intra-abdominal surgery and diverticulosis has simple incomplete small-bowel obstruction (without compromised blood flow) and has had nausea and vomiting for 2 days. Which of the following initial interventions are most indicated?

    a. Immediate surgical repair.
    b. Nasogastric (NG) decompression and IV fluids.
    c. NG decompression and antibiotic therapy.
    d. NG decompression only.

72. An 18-year-old patient became angry at her parents and ingested 10,000 mg of extra-strength acetaminophen and was found by her mother 12 hours later. The patient was pale, nauseated, and diaphoretic but had not vomited. The AGACNP should recognize that the patient is at risk for:

    a. renal failure.
    b. liver failure.
    c. intestinal obstruction.
    d. gastrointestinal (GI) bleeding.

73. If the AGACNP is newly hired at a healthcare organization and believes that there is a need for improvement in patient care, the first thing the AGACNP should assess is the:

    a. workplace culture.
    b. available resources.
    c. knowledge base of the staff.
    d. administrative support.

74. If the AGACNP notes that a patient's blood pressure has fallen precipitously and the pulse rate has increased but fails to take action and the patient suffers permanent injury as a result, the element of malpractice that applies to the AGACNP is:

    a. causation.
    b. foreseeability.
    c. breach of duty owed.
    d. duty owed to the patient.

75. A patient with ptosis and extraocular weakness with a presumed diagnosis of myasthenia gravis is undergoing the Tensilon (edrophonium chloride) challenge. With a positive finding, the patient exhibits:

    a. worsening ptosis and weakening.
    b. improvement in ptosis and weakening.
    c. no change in ptosis and weakening.
    d. muscular twitching of the eyelid.

76. If a patient comes to the emergency department vomiting bright-red blood and is hemodynamically unstable, the initial response should be to type and crossmatch for packed red blood cells and to:

    a. administer 2 to 3 units of type O packed red blood cells.
    b. administer 0.9% saline or lactated Ringer's solution.
    c. insert a nasogastric tube.
    d. carry out gastric lavage.

77. The AGACNP has instituted staff rounding with a goal of meeting with each staff member at least once weekly. The purpose of staff rounding is to:

    a. update staff members on changes and/or needs.
    b. discuss the staff members' performance issues.
    c. improve communication and support staff members' needs.
    d. eliminate small problems before they become large.

78. The AGACNP has taught a patient's spouse to change the patient's dressing and to understand signs of healing and infection. The best method to ensure that the patient's spouse is able to carry out the dressing change and monitor the wound is to ask for a

    a. written test.
    b. verbal description of the procedure.
    c. return demonstration.
    d. follow-up wound assessment.

79. A patient has acute nongonococcal bacterial (septic) arthritis of the knee. Immediate treatment includes antibiotics and:

    a. drainage of the joint.
    b. hot compresses.
    c. cold compresses.
    d. nonsteroidal anti-inflammatory drugs (NSAIDs).

80. A 32-year-old patient suffered carbon monoxide (CO) toxicity and is receiving 100% oxygen per nonrebreather mask. The patient should be maintained on 100% oxygen therapy until the patient is asymptomatic and the hemoglobin CO level falls to less than:

    a. 20%.
    b. 10%.
    c. 5%.
    d. 2%.

81. If a 73-year-old patient is admitted from a residential care facility with a coccygeal pressure ulcer that is 6 cm by 4 cm and extends to the muscle and is partially covered with black necrotic tissue, the AGACNP would classify the pressure ulcer with National Pressure Ulcer Advisory Panel (NPUAP) staging as:

    a. Stage I.
    b. Stage II.
    c. Stage III.
    d. Stage IV.

82. The AGACNP intends to implement a new procedure in the delivery of patient care, understanding that the biggest threat to implementation of change is usually:

    a. staff resistance.
    b. lack of adequate preparation.
    c. poor change design.
    d. insufficient supporting data.

83. The AGACNP overhears another nurse complaining that an adult female Hmong patient is subservient and dependent because she allows her father to make decisions about her health care and that the nurse tried without success to convince the patient to make her own decisions. This type of intervention would best be described as:

    a. ethnocentrism.
    b. cultural imposition.
    c. stereotyping.
    d. cultural competence.

84. A 21-year-old African-American female presents with a malar rash, Raynaud's phenomenon, joint pain and stiffness, positive antinuclear antibody (ANA), and thrombocytopenia of 90,000/mcL. Based on these findings, the probable diagnosis is:

    a. systemic lupus erythematosus.
    b. rheumatoid arthritis.
    c. adult Still disease.
    d. scleroderma.

85. When the AGACNP is assessing a patient with neurological injury, which of the following indicates an upper motor neuron lesion?

    a. Muscle spasticity.
    b. Muscle flaccidity.
    c. Muscle atrophy.
    d. Absent reflexes.

86. A 66-year-old patient with a history of alcoholic cirrhosis has developed small esophageal varices but no bleeding. Which of the following preventive treatments is most appropriate?

    a. Shunt surgery.
    b. Nitrate.
    c. Sclerotherapy.
    d. Nonselective beta-blocker.

87. If a 25-year-old patient's body mass index (BMI) is 17.5 and the albumin level is normal at 3.8 g/dL (38 g/L) (normal value is 3.5 to 5.5 g/dL OR 35 to 55 g/L) and prealbumin shows moderate deficiency of 6 mg/dL (60 mg/L) (normal is 16 to 40 mg/dL OR 160 to 400 mg/L), these findings suggest:

    a. long-term protein malnutrition.
    b. short-term protein malnutrition.
    c. adequate protein but inadequate calories.
    d. adequate calories but inadequate protein.

88. The AGACNP has proposed use of the Situation-Background-Assessment-Recommendation (SBAR) format for hand-off communication but is encountering resistance from long-time staff members who dislike change. The best method of dealing with resistance is to:

    a. ignore the complaints.
    b. inform resistant staff members that they are impeding the process.
    c. encourage staff to express opinions and discuss concerns.
    d. propose a vote regarding the use of SBAR.

89. If the AGACNP hears a patient's physician complaining that a patient is "difficult and impatient," and the AGACNP tells the physician that the patient is very frightened and acting defensively, the aspect of care that the AGACNP is exhibiting is:

    a. advocacy.
    b. patient equality.
    c. human dignity preservation.
    e. caring practice.

90. In the event of a disaster, which initial strategy could be employed to increase a hospital's surge capacity?

    a. Identify clients safely eligible for early discharge.
    b. Place extra beds in private rooms.
    c. Recommend closing the emergency department to non-disaster-related clients.
    d. Transfer clients so that open rooms are in close proximity.

91. Which of the following is a correct presentation of a medication order in an electronic health record (EHR) with a medication order set?

    a. Penicillin G 6,000,000 U I.V. every 4 hours.
    b. ASA 325 mg qd.
    c. 112 µg levothyroxine daily.
    d. Paroxetine hydrochloride 20 mg P.O. daily in AM.

92. When confidential patient data are contained on mobile devices, such as smartphones or personal digital assistants (PDAs), these devices should:

    a. contain locking and tracking software.
    b. not leave a secure facility.
    c. be used by only one person.
    d. contain only de-identified health information.

93. If a patient has been diagnosed with tuberculosis (TB), how long does the first-line drug susceptibility testing (liquid medium) take before results are available?

    a. 24 hours.
    b. 24 to 48 hours.
    c. 1 to 2 weeks.
    d. 3 to 4 weeks.

94. Under the Joint Commission's National Patient Safety Goals, which of the following is generally acceptable as one of two required identifiers?

    a. Place of birth.
    b. Date of birth.
    c. Place of employment.
    d. Verifying patient's name from armband taped to bedside stand.

95. When an insurance plan negotiates a specific fee for a procedure (including all charges) and pays one bill, this is referred to as:

    a. unbundling.
    b. bundling.
    c. fee-for-service.
    d. discounted fee-for-service.

96. A 25-year-old patient has developed itchy, red, sharply defined, scaly lesions in both axillae. Which of the following additional finding supports a diagnosis of psoriasis?

    a. Low-grade fever.
    b. Obesity with BMI >31.
    c. Elevated WBC count.
    d. Fine stippling of the fingernails.

97. In order to receive Medicare reimbursement for coverage of nurse practitioner services, the services must be:

    a. provided subject to state restrictions and supervision requirements.
    b. provided under direct supervision.
    c. provided in a rural health clinic (RHC) or federally qualified health center (FQHC).
    d. billed through a physician-directed clinic, health agency, or hospital.

98. According to Knowles' principles of adult learning, adult learners tend to be:

    a. unmotivated.
    b. lacking in self-direction.
    c. practical and goal-oriented.
    d. insecure.

99. The ethnic group that has the highest prevalence of asthma is:

    a. Caucasian.
    b. African-American.
    c. Asian.
    d. Polynesian.

100. Which of the following Healthcare Common Procedure Coding System (HCPCS) level II codes is used when filing a Medicare claim for durable medical equipment, such as a bedside commode?

    a. D codes.
    b. E codes.
    c. L codes.
    d. P codes.

101. One week after a tick bite, a patient develops erythema migrans (15 cm diameter) (a bull's-eye rash) with slight burning at the bite site. In an area endemic to Lyme disease, the treatment of choice is:

 a. azithromycin 500 mg for 3 days.
 b. erythromycin 500 mg BID for 7 days.
 c. ciprofloxacin 500 mg BID for 1 to 2 weeks.
 d. doxycycline 100 mg BID for 2 to 3 weeks.

102. The Health Insurance Portability and Accountability Act of 1996 (HIPAA) Security Rule applies to protected health information (PHI) that is transmitted:

 a. orally.
 b. in writing.
 c. electronically.
 d. in any manner.

103. Which of the following is typically present with vertigo associated with Ménière's syndrome?

 a. tinnitus and low-frequency hearing loss.
 b. headache.
 c. photosensitivity.
 d. head pressure.

104. Health literacy is directly affected by general literacy, so when educating patients, the AGACNP should realize that the approximate percentage of adults in the U.S. who are classified as illiterate or low literate is:

 a. 25%.
 b. 40%.
 c. 50%.
 d. 70%.

105. A 72-year-old patient has three polyps removed during a routine colonoscopy. Which of the following types of polyps are precancerous?

 a. Epithelial hyperplastic.
 b. Adenomatous.
 c. Inflammatory.
 d. Submucosal (fibroma).

106. Female patients should generally be advised to begin breast cancer screening with routine mammograms at about age:

 a. 20 to 30.
 b. 30 to 40.
 c. 40 to 50.
 d. 50 to 60.

107. Which of the following conditions of the breast may pose the greatest risk for the development of breast cancer?

 a. Lipoma.
 b. Hemangioma.
 c. Epithelial-related calcifications.
 d. Atypical ductal hyperplasia.

- 82 -

108. Which of the following healthcare services can an adolescent younger than 18 access or refuse without parental knowledge or consent in most states?

    a. emergency contraception.
    b. abortion.
    c. chemotherapy.
    d. transfusions.

109. The AGACNP has prescribed acetaminophen for a 78-year-old patient and should advise the patient to limit total dosage to:

    a. 1 g in 24 hours.
    b. 2 g in 24 hours.
    c. 3 g in 24 hours.
    d. 4 g in 24 hours.

110. The patient's problem list contains the following four items: (1) hypertension (150/92), (2) diabetes mellitus, type 2 (A1C 8%), (3) neuropathy of both feet, and (4) infected ingrown toenail. Treatment would be prioritized (ranked from highest priority to lowest):

    a. 4, 2, 1, and 3.
    b. 2, 4, 1, and 3.
    c. 1, 2, 4, and 3.
    d. 2, 1, 3, and 4.

111. The AGACNP is educating a patient who is to be discharged after surgery to remove a cancerous lesion of the colon and create a colostomy. The AGACNP advises the patient that foods that may cause a noticeable odor include:

    a. green beans, raw fruits, spicy foods, and spinach.
    b. popcorn, seeds, raw vegetables, and corn.
    c. fish, eggs, onions, broccoli, asparagus, and cabbage.
    d. beans, carbonated beverages, strong cheeses, and sprouts.

112. If an Orthodox Jewish male patient needs an examination, and the AGACNP is female, the AGACNP should:

    a. ask the patient if he would prefer to be examined by a male nurse.
    b. carry out the examination unless the patient complains.
    c. refuse to examine the patient.
    d. only ask questions but avoid touching the patient.

113. When collecting a medication history, the AGACNP should include:

    a. prescription drugs only.
    b. prescription drugs and over-the-counter (OTC) drugs.
    c. prescription drugs, OTC drugs, and vitamin supplements.
    d. prescription drugs, OTC drugs, vitamin supplements, and any other health-related substance.

114. Which class of medications should be avoided in frail elderly adults?

    a. Nonsteroidal anti-inflammatory drugs (NSAIDs).
    b. Benzodiazepines.
    c. Beta-blockers.
    d. Bronchodilators.

115. If a patient who appears to be a drug seeker demands a prescription for OxyContin for severe chronic migraine headaches, the best response is likely to:

a. believe the patient.
b. provide a small amount of drugs.
c. verify the patient's medical history with previous healthcare providers.
d. refuse service to the patient.

116. If a patient telephones the acute care telehealth line with complaints of abdominal pain and the AGACNP is screening the patient, which of the following additional symptoms represents an emergent situation and should result in the AGACNP advising the patient to hang up and call 9-1-1?

a. Fever of 38°C/100.4°F and slight chills.
b. Increasing shortness of breath and chest discomfort.
c. Severe constipation for 2 to 3 days.
d. Mild nausea and vomiting twice in 24 hours.

117. A 22-year-old female patient who is nulliparous and sexually active with multiple sex partners presents in the emergency department with chills and a temperature of 39°C, purulent vaginal discharge, lower abdominal pain, and cervical and adnexal tenderness. Ectopic pregnancy is ruled out. Based on these findings, the patient should receive treatment for probable:

a. pelvic inflammatory disease.
b. cervicitis.
c. endometriosis.
d. bacterial vaginosis.

118. Which of the following hematology tests is outside of normal parameters for an adult male?

a. Red blood cell (RBC) count of 4.6 million/mm³.
b. Hemoglobin (Hgb) of 15 g/dL.
c. Hematocrit (Hct) of 44%.
d. White blood cell (WBC) count of 4100/mm³.

119. A patient with stage 4 prostate cancer has recently completed a course of radiation to relieve spinal compression from bone metastasis. His pain is well controlled with Fentanyl, but he is fearful and he has developed tremors and jerking movements of his extremities, and these are keeping him awake at night. The most likely cause of the tremor and jerking movements is:

a. brain metastasis.
b. spinal damage.
c. anxiety.
d. opioid-induced myoclonus.

120. When the AGACNP enters the room of a patient whose death is imminent, the daughter states, "I can't stay in the room when Dad dies! I can't stand the thought!" The best response is:

a. "You will regret it if you don't."
b. "Your father would want you with him."
c. "I'll stay with him, and you can come and go as you feel comfortable."
d. "Is there someone else who can stay with him?"

121. A patient with ovarian cancer suddenly develops severe nausea and vomiting in large volumes. Her abdomen is painful and rigid, her bowel sounds are diminished, and she feels short of breath. She has no fever. She reports that she has had only very small bowel movements recently. The most likely diagnosis is:

a. fecal impaction.
b. obstruction of small intestines.
c. obstruction of colon.
d. peritonitis.

122. A 32-year-old male presents with swelling, erythema, and severe pain of the metatarsophalangeal (MTP) joint of the right great toe after a night of excessive drinking. Lab testing shows elevated uric acid, confirming an acute gout attack. The most appropriate treatment is:

a. a nonsteroidal anti-inflammatory drug (NSAID).
b. colchicine.
c. a corticosteroid.
d. an antibiotic.

123. A patient has marked bilateral nonpitting edema of both lower legs and feet, including his toes, and he has thickening of the skin but no pigmentation. This edema can most likely be characterized as:

a. orthostatic edema.
b. lymphedema.
c. lipedema.
d. chronic venous insufficiency.

124. Which of the following is the correct documentation of undermining?

a. "Extends 1.8 cm width about one-quarter of the wound perimeter."
b. "Extends ¾ inch width by the right lower quadrant of the wound."
c. "Extends 1.8 cm width from 1 o'clock to 4 o'clock."
d. "Extends ¾ inch width from 1 o'clock to 4 o'clock."

125. If, while conducting a peer review, the AGACNP observes the other nurse using nontherapeutic communication techniques with a patient, the best response is to:

a. immediately intervene.
b. discuss at a post-review meeting.
c. report the observation to a supervisor.
d. ignore it because it does not constitute negligence.

126. The four nonverbal behaviors that are associated with active listening include:

a. sit beside the patient, maintain open posture, lean back comfortably, and maintain eye contact.
b. sit across from the patient, maintain closed posture, lean forward, and avoid eye contact.
c. sit across from the patient, maintain open posture, lean forward, and maintain eye contact.
d. sit beside the patient, maintain open posture, lean forward, and maintain eye contact.

127. A 20-year-old patient with Tourette's syndrome has had increasing social problems and academic problems, often having difficulty completing activities. For which common comorbidity should the patient be evaluated?

a. Obsessive-compulsive disorder (OCD).
b. Depression.
c. Schizophrenia.
d. Bipolar disorder.

128. A 16-year-old patient identifying as a girl fails to begin menstruation despite breast development and develops only scant pubic and underarm hair. On physical examination, the patient is found to have only a vaginal stump but no cervix or uterus, and inguinal testes are found. Testing shows that the patient is genetically male and has complete androgen insensitivity syndrome (CAIS). The best approach with the patient is to:

a. provide the information only to the parents.
b. advise the patient to transition to living as a male.
c. withhold the information until the patient is 18.
d. provide a full explanation to the patient.

129. When screening an older adult for depression with the Geriatric Depression Scale, short form (GDS-SF) with 15 questions, what is the minimal score that indicates possible depression?

a. 3
b. 6
c. 8
d. 10

130. During registration, a new patient must sign an assignment of benefits form so that the:

a. patient can receive reimbursement for claims.
b. provider is prohibited from releasing information about the patient.
c. provider can have access to the healthcare record.
d. provider can bill the insurance companies.

131. A 32-year-old woman with autoimmune myasthenia gravis (MG) has fluctuating but increasing muscle weakness. She reports that she has begun to sleep in her chair because she sleeps better sitting upright, and during the interview, she yawns and sighs frequently. Which of the following interventions is most appropriate based on these symptoms?

a. Respiratory assessment with pulmonary function tests.
b. Acetylcholine receptor (AChR) antibody titer.
c. Repetitive nerve stimulation.
d. Ice pack test.

132. A 74-year-old woman recovering from hip surgery had been mentally alert prior to surgery but has a sudden change in mental status with disorientation, fluctuations in level of consciousness, and agitation. Her medications include Glucophage, a thiazide diuretic, and acetaminophen with codeine. Which of the following is the most appropriate initial intervention for suspected delirium?

a. Provide side rails and restraints to prevent injury.
b. Provide antipsychotic medication to control symptoms.
c. Ask the patient to count backward from 20 to 1 to assess attention.
d. Discontinue all medications immediately.

133. Parenteral nutrition with a total nutrient admixture (TNA) that includes lipids has been ordered for a burn patient for administration over a 24-hour period. When preparing to administer the solution, the AGACNP observes that the oil has separated, forming an obvious layer. Which is the correct action?

    a. Administer the solution because oil separation is normal.
    b. Mix the solution by shaking the bag until no oil separation is noticeable.
    c. Discard the solution.
    d. Return the solution to the pharmacy for addition of an emulsifier.

134. Ensuring that a patient has given informed consent and understands his or her rights and all of the risks and benefits of a procedure or treatment supports the ethical principle of:

    a. beneficence.
    b. nonmaleficence.
    c. justice.
    d. autonomy.

135. A 24-year-old patient was diagnosed with type 1 diabetes mellitus after presenting with a glucose level of 468 mg/dL (26 mmol/L), polyuria, polydipsia, and weight loss. His condition has stabilized since starting insulin injections, and the patient now appears to be able to manage the diabetes with very little insulin. The AGACNP should suspect that the:

    a. patient's insulin needs will increase again.
    b. patient will no longer need to take insulin.
    c. patient was misdiagnosed and has type 2 diabetes.
    d. patient's condition will remain stable at this level.

136. A 16-year-old adolescent is being treated with fluoxetine (a selective serotonin reuptake inhibitor [SSRI]) and cognitive behavioral therapy (CBT) for severe anxiety and depression 6 months after the death of her mother. The girl must be monitored and regularly assessed for:

    a. substance abuse.
    b. polypharmacy.
    c. suicidal ideation.
    d. noncompliance.

137. Which of the following is an example of therapeutic communication?

    a. "You should try not to worry."
    b. "Don't worry. Everything will be fine."
    c. "Why are you so upset?"
    d. "I'd like to hear how you feel about that."

138. A 72-year-old female on Medicare is being discharged home with a healing burn on her left arm that she is unable to care for independently because of arthritis. She requires dressing changes every 3 days. She depends on public transportation and walks with difficulty. The bus stop is two blocks from her house. Her 12-year-old granddaughter lives with her. The best solution is:

    a. transferring the patient to an extended care facility.
    b. providing treatment on an outpatient basis at the hospital clinic.
    c. teaching the woman's 12-year-old granddaughter to do the dressing changes.
    d. making a referral to a home health agency to provide in-home care.

139. A patient has a long leg cast and requires assessment to ensure the cast is not restrictive. The 5 Ps of neurovascular assessment include (1) pain, (2) pallor, (3) pulselessness, (4) paresthesia, and (5):

    a. Paraplegia.
    b. Pallesthesia.
    c. Paralysis.
    d. Pathology.

140. A 42-year-old woman is receiving end-of-life care for stage 4 breast cancer. She has developed a pronounced bronchial death rattle, which is very distressing to her adolescent daughter and son. Death is expected within a few hours. Which of the following treatments is most indicated to relieve the death rattle?

    a. Glycopyrrolate or atropine subcutaneously (subQ).
    b. Morphine sulfate subQ.
    c. Hyoscine hydrobromide (scopolamine) transdermal patch.
    d. Oropharyngeal suctioning.

141. A 68-year-old male has an asynchronous pacemaker and has been experiencing cardiac palpitations, headache, and anxiety, general malaise, pain in the jaw and chest, and unexplained weakness with pulsations evident in the neck and abdomen. The most likely cause is:

    a. broken pacemaker wires.
    b. dislodging of pacemaker wires.
    c. myocardial infarction.
    d. pacemaker syndrome.

142. Using the average cost of a problem and the cost of intervention to demonstrate savings is a(n):

    a. cost-benefit analysis.
    b. efficacy study.
    c. product evaluation.
    d. cost-effectiveness analysis.

143. A retrospective attempt to determine the cause of an event, often a sentinel event such as an unexpected death, is:

    a. the *t*-test.
    b. regression analysis.
    c. the tracer methodology.
    d. root cause analysis.

144. A 62-year-old patient is diagnosed with active pulmonary tuberculosis (TB). Active pulmonary TB is characterized by which of the following?

    a. High fever, cough, diaphoresis.
    b. Fatigue, high fever, weight gain.
    c. Chest pain, diaphoresis, malaise.
    d. Night sweats, cough, low-grade fever.

145. As leader of an interdisciplinary team, the AGACNP notes that one team member who has worked on the unit for more than 20 years frequently criticizes younger and less experienced nurses. The best initial approach to resolve this is to:

    a. ask the experienced nurse to serve as a mentor.

    b. ask the experienced nurse to be more patient and supportive.

    c. tell the experienced nurse that the behavior is detrimental to the team.

    d. suggest that the experienced nurse transfer to a different team.

146. The three elements that the Quality and Safety Education for Nurses (QSEN) initiative focus on include (1) knowledge, (2) skills, and (3):

    a. roles.

    b. attitudes.

    c. certification.

    d. responsibilities.

147. If a patient is prescribed five different medications, the chance for drug interactions because of polypharmacy is approximately:

    a. 10%.

    b. 25%.

    c. 50%.

    d. 100%.

148. A 36-year-old woman comes to the emergency department complaining of vaginal discharge that started two days prior to the expected onset of menstruation. The findings consistent with vaginal candidiasis include:

    a. vaginal pain and purulent discharge.

    b. vaginal itching and watery, foul-smelling discharge.

    c. urinary frequency, vaginal pain, and foul-smelling discharge.

    d. vaginal itching and thick, white, adherent discharge.

149. The AGACNP has been teaching an Asian patient how to manage her diabetes, including taking blood glucose readings and administering insulin. However, the patient asks no questions, and when the AGACNP asks the patient if she understands, the patient always says "Yes," even though she seems quite confused with the procedures. The primary problem probably is:

    a. the patient is too confused to respond appropriately.

    b. the patient's response is culturally different from what the nurse expects.

    c. the patient doesn't want to hurt the nurse's feelings.

    d. the patient is afraid of the nurse.

150. Cushing's triad (hypertension, bradycardia, and widening pulse pressure) in patients with increased intracranial pressure from a traumatic brain injury may be a sign of:

    a. brain herniation.

    b. subdural hematoma.

    c. impending seizures.

    d. cerebral infection.

151. Fifteen hours after a patient was involved in an automobile accident, the patient presents in the emergency department with abdominal discomfort and a positive Cullen's sign (bruising about the umbilicus). The AGACNP should suspect:

    a. ruptured spleen.
    b. retroperitoneal bleeding.
    c. hepatic laceration.
    d. ruptured diaphragm.

152. The first step in diagnosing an acid-base disturbance is to:

    a. evaluate pCO_2.
    b. evaluate HCO_3.
    c. evaluate pO_2.
    d. evaluate pH.

153. If using the PQRST method to assess a patient's chest pain (**P**recipitating events, **Q**uality of pain/discomfort, **R**adiation of pain, **S**everity of pain, and **T**...), the "T" stand for:

    a. timing.
    b. tachycardia.
    c. temperature.
    d. transmission.

154. Following gastric bypass surgery that includes removal of the pyloric valve, dumping syndrome is often precipitated by:

    a. high-protein diets.
    b. overeating.
    c. high-sugar (carbohydrate) foods.
    d. fatty foods.

155. When examining a patient's breasts for masses, the AGACNP is aware that the most common site for breast cancer is in the:

    a. upper medial quadrant of the breast.
    b. upper lateral quadrant of the breast.
    c. lower medial quadrant of the breast.
    d. lower lateral quadrant of the breast.

156. About 70% of cervical cancer cases are linked to a history of:

    a. human immunodeficiency virus (HIV) infection.
    b. obesity.
    c. multiparity.
    d. human papilloma virus (HPV).

157. The AGACNP overhears a nurse complain that if the hospital treats an uninsured homeless patient, it will be overwhelmed with many more homeless patients and go bankrupt. What type of logical fallacy does this represent?

    a. Slippery slope.
    b. Overgeneralization.
    c. Post hoc.
    d. Hasty generalization.

158. A patient who has taken opioids for pain for a prolonged period complains that the drugs are less effective. The adaptive state in which the effects of opioid drugs diminish over time is:

    a. physical dependence.
    b. psychological dependence.
    c. opioid tolerance.
    d. drug interaction.

159. If a patient with a head injury has a slightly elevated intracranial pressure (ICP) but develops a high fever, the AGACNP expects the fever to:

    a. decrease ICP and cerebral perfusion pressure (CPP).
    b. increase ICP and CPP.
    c. increase ICP and decrease CPP.
    d. decrease ICP and increase CPP.

160. Which of the following heart conditions results in stiffened heart muscles that cannot contract adequately?

    a. Myocarditis.
    b. Hypertrophic cardiomyopathy.
    c. Dilated cardiomyopathy.
    d. Restrictive cardiomyopathy.

161. Which of the following should be screened for hepatitis C?

    a. Adults born from 1945 through 1965.
    b. All patients with kidney disease.
    c. Anyone who received blood after 1992.
    d. All healthcare workers.

162. Which of the following findings on a urinalysis may indicate a urinary tract infection?

    a. SpGr 1.020.
    b. Urobilinogen 0.4 units.
    c. Glucose, negative.
    d. pH 8.1

163. If a patient is on the National Dysphagia Diet 1 (NND1 Dysphagia—pureed) diet, which of the following foods would be excluded?

    a. Scrambled eggs.
    b. Pureed meats.
    c. Mashed potatoes.
    d. Ice cream.

164. Which of the following findings indicates that a patient needs an X-ray to evaluate a probable fractured knee?

    a. Inability to flex more than 90°.
    b. Inability to take four steps or bear weight.
    c. Limping when walking.
    d. Swelling around the knee.

165. A patient with rheumatoid arthritis (RA) complains of dry eyes, dry mouth, dry lips, and increasing dysphagia. The extra-articular manifestation of RA that the AGACNP should suspect is:

    a. Caplan syndrome.
    b. Felty syndrome.
    c. Sjogren's syndrome.
    d. Amyloidosis.

166. A 60-year-old female patient diagnosed with nonalcoholic fatty liver disease is obese and has metabolic syndrome. The AGACNP should advise the patient to:

    a. Gradually lose 10% of body weight.
    b. Avoid all alcohol.
    c. Rapidly lose at least 20 pounds.
    d. Restrict sodium and fluid intake.

167. If the AGACNP is sexually harassed by a member of the medical staff in an episode witnessed by three coworkers, but the coworkers say they do not want to be involved when the AGACNP documents the harassment in an incident report, the most appropriate action is to:

    a. not file the incident report.
    b. file the incident report with no reference to witnesses.
    c. file the incident report and list witnesses.
    d. complain to a supervisor without documenting the incident.

168. A 38-year-old male patient comes to the emergency department with severe left flank pain from a kidney stone. The priority treatment should be to:

    a. strain the urine.
    b. administer analgesia.
    c. increase hydration.
    d. administer a beta-blocker.

169. A patient with a history of alcoholism complains of problems with sleep. Which of the following is true about alcohol and sleep disturbance?

    a. Patients tend to sleep more at night but are sleepy during the daytime.
    b. Sleep is severely disrupted, and patients may only sleep for short periods.
    c. Patients experience adequate total sleep time but inadequate rapid eye-movement (REM) sleep.
    d. Sedation occurs early with acute intoxication but is later replaced with increased wakefulness and restlessness.

170. For which type of wound is hydrotherapy contraindicated?

    a. Burns.
    b. Cancerous wound.
    c. Venous ulcers.
    d. Infectious wound.

171. Which of the following topical medications may be prescribed to treat a patient's burns and is effective against Gram-positive organisms?

    a. Silver sulfadiazine.
    b. Cadexomer iodine.
    c. Polymyxin B.
    d. Mupirocin.

172. Which of the following dressing types should the AGACNP advise for a full-thickness necrotic wound with a small amount of exudate?

    a. Hydrocolloid.
    b. Hydrogel.
    c. Alginate.
    d. Foam.

173. Because of the high incidence of comorbidity, a patient who has been diagnosed with Addison's disease (primary adrenal insufficiency) should be screened for:

    a. aortic aneurysm.
    b. diabetes mellitus.
    c. lactose intolerance.
    d. celiac disease.

174. If a patient is hospitalized with Guillain-Barré syndrome, the treatment of choice is:

    a. broad-spectrum antibiotics.
    b. corticosteroids.
    c. plasmapheresis or immunoglobulin therapy.
    d. methotrexate.

175. Patients with long-term urinary catheters are at high risk of developing resistant infections because of:

    a. development of biofilms in the bladder.
    b. development of bladder ulcerations.
    c. trauma related to catheter movement.
    d. blockage of urinary catheters.

176. In the ABCDEs of melanoma, *E* refers to:

    a. ecchymosis.
    b. enlargement.
    c. emerging lesion.
    d. evolving changes.

177. Patients who have sickle cell disease receive hydroxyurea to:

    a. treat iron deficiency anemia.
    b. decrease sickling.
    c. prevent infection.
    d. prevent dehydration.

178. The AGACNP should warn a patient who is prescribed varenicline (Chantix) for nicotine dependence to be alert for:

    a. psychiatric symptoms/suicidal ideation.
    b. skin irritation and itching.
    c. excessive drowsiness.
    d. nausea, vomiting, and diarrhea.

179. As part of stroke rehabilitation, the primary purpose of functional electrical stimulation devices is to:

    a. prevent muscular atrophy.
    b. trigger sensory responses.
    c. improve functional ability.
    d. record muscle activity.

180. A patient on hemodialysis has an arteriovenous fistula in the right forearm. If the patient requires a blood draw, the blood should be drawn:

    a. from the arteriovenous fistula.
    b. distal to the arteriovenous fistula.
    c. proximal to the arteriovenous fistula.
    d. from the left arm.

181. If a patient complains of sudden-onset "tearing" chest pain associated with severe back pain, the AGACNP should suspect that the origin of the pain is:

    a. an aortic dissection.
    b. a pulmonary embolism.
    c. cardiovascular ischemia.
    d. the gastrointestinal (GI) system.

182. An 80-year-old patient with peripheral arterial disease states he has severe pain in the dorsum and toes of the right foot and toes when lying in bed at night, but the pain is relieved somewhat when he stands up. These symptoms indicate possible:

    a. vascular spasms.
    b. increasing neuropathy.
    c. critical limb ischemia.
    d. intermittent claudication.

183. A patient with multiple sclerosis (MS) has shown steady progression of the disease since diagnosis but has periodic episodes of acute exacerbations and remissions. This type of MS is classified as:

    a. Relapsing-remitting.
    b. Progressive relapsing.
    c. Primary progressive.
    d. Secondary progressive.

184. A patient asks the AGACNP about the feasibility of traveling to a high elevation (higher than 13,000 feet) in the mountains of Colorado to stay with family members after discharge from the hospital. Which of the following conditions would preclude such travel?

  a. Diabetes mellitus.
  b. Hypertension
  c. Human immunodeficiency virus/acquired immunodeficiency syndrome (HIV/AIDS).
  d. Sickle cell disease.

185. A patient who has been intubated for 3 days is now breathing independently and is to begin oral fluids. The initial action should be to:

  a. carry out a bedside swallowing test.
  b. offer the patient ice cubes to suck on.
  c. begin with warm fluids, such as broth.
  d. ask the patient for fluid preference.

186. If a patient has a proximal small-bowel obstruction with abdominal pain and distension, the AGACNP likely also documents:

  a. abdominal pain and distension only.
  b. nausea and dry heaves but no vomiting.
  c. rapid onset of nausea and projectile vomiting of bile emesis.
  d. gradual onset of nausea and vomiting of orange-brown, fecal-smelling emesis.

187. A homeless patient was admitted to the emergency department with an open venous stasis ulcer, which was covered with maggots, on the lower legs. The maggots likely:

  a. infected the ulcer.
  b. debrided the ulcer.
  c. expanded the ulcer.
  d. had no effect on the ulcer.

188. The AGACNP asks the patient to stick out the tongue and examines the thrust for symmetry and then asks the patient to say "light, tight, dynamite." The cranial nerve that the AGACNP is evaluating is:

  a. cranial nerve IX.
  b. cranial nerve X.
  c. cranial nerve XI.
  d. cranial nerve XII.

189. A 40-year-old patient with Huntington's disease, an autosomal dominant disorder, has three children. What percentage chance does each child have of inheriting the disorder?

  a. 25%.
  b. 50%.
  c. 75%.
  d. 100%.

190. A 34-year-old patient with schizophrenia was maintained on antipsychotic drugs but stopped taking the medications and is hospitalized with both positive and negative symptoms. An example of a negative symptom is:

    a. flat affect.
    b. hallucination.
    c. delusion.
    d. catatonic behavior.

191. The standard triple therapy for *Helicobacter pylori*-associated peptic ulcer disease includes a proton pump inhibitor two times a day (BID), clarithromycin 500 mg BID, and:

    a. bismuth subcitrate potassium 140 mg qd.
    b. an H_2 receptor antagonist.
    c. amoxicillin 1 g BID.
    d. misoprostol 200 mcg QID.

192. Immigrants from which of the following countries are most at risk of having Chagas disease?

    a. Brazil.
    b. Mexico.
    c. Philippines.
    d. Vietnam.

193. Symptoms that are common to patients with a tumor in the cerebellum include:

    a. changes in mood and personality.
    b. lack of coordination and balance.
    c. visual and auditory hallucinations.
    d. blurred vision and diplopia.

194. Following a bout of West Nile Fever, the symptom that is likely to persist for the longest period is:

    a. fatigue.
    b. headache.
    c. fever.
    d. muscle weakness.

195. A patient has returned from a trip to Africa with symptoms of malaria. The classic cycle of symptoms for uncomplicated malaria include:

    a. headache stage, fever, stage, chill stage.
    b. fever stage, jaundice stage, and hepatosplenomegaly stage.
    c. headache stage, fever stage, nausea stage.
    d. cold stage, hot stage, sweating stage.

196. Medications that can cause an increased risk of osteoporosis include:

    a. corticosteroids.
    b. bisphosphonates.
    c. beta blockers.
    d. fluoroquinolones.

197. If a patient is hospitalized with heat exhaustion, how much of the total water depletion should be replaced with rehydration within the first 3 to 6 hours?

 a. 100%.
 b. 75%.
 c. 50%.
 d. 25%.

198. A patient is experiencing an acute episode of asthma and is anxious, sitting in the tripod position with audible wheezing resulting from an upper airway obstruction. The patient's peak flow is 65% of normal, and oxygen saturation is 92%. The initial rescue protocol should begin with:

 a. albuterol.
 b. prednisone or methylprednisolone.
 c. an antihistamine, such as diphenhydramine.
 d. theophylline.

199. Which of the following drugs are less effective for treating hypertension in African-American patients?

 a. Angiotensin-converting enzyme (ACE) inhibitors and angiotensin II receptor blockers (ARBs).
 b. Beta-blockers and diuretics.
 c. Diuretics and calcium channel blockers.
 d. Calcium channel blockers and ACE inhibitors.

200. With the timed up and go (TUG) test to assess ambulation and mobility, which completion time indicates an increased risk for falls?

 a. 10 seconds.
 b. 8 seconds.
 c. 14 seconds.
 d. 5 seconds.

Answers and Explanations

1. C: For patients with diabetes mellitus, the first indication of diabetic nephropathy, the most common cause of end-stage renal disease, is usually microalbuminuria. Microalbuminuria is usually detectable before a decrease in the glomerular filtration rate (GFR) and occurs 10 to 15 years after the onset of diabetes. With the onset of microalbuminuria, the patient should be maintained on strict glycemic control and treatment of hypertension to slow the progression. Angiotensin-converting enzyme (ACE) inhibitors and angiotensin II receptor blockers (ARBs) have been shown to slow progression by reducing pressure within the glomeruli.

2. D: If a 36-year-old male patient has acute sexually transmitted epididymitis, in addition to antibiotics during the acute phase of the disease, the treatment regimen should include bed rest and scrotal elevation, which may help to alleviate some of the pain. Treatment usually continues for 10 to 21 days. Sexually transmitted epididymitis is most common in males younger than age 40. Laboratory findings include elevated white blood cell (WBC) count and left shift. Gram stain may be done to isolate the pathogen for sexually transmitted disease.

3. B: When a patient, such as a burn patient, is placed on an air-fluidized bed, it is especially important to monitor fluid balance because he or she can easily become dehydrated. Air-fluidized beds contain a mass of fine ceramic microspheres through which warm air flows. The patient is placed on a special polyester filter sheet that allows air to pass through it. The warmth causes perspiration, which is quickly absorbed, so diaphoresis may not be evident.

4. A: At a body mass index (BMI) of ≥30, patients are considered obese and should be counseled regarding diet, lifestyle choice, and weight loss goals. The body mass index (BMI) is based on weight and height:

- Weight (kg) ÷ (height)^2 (m) = BMI.
- Weight (lb) ÷ [height (in)]^2 × 703 = BMI.

BMI	Weight status
<18.5	Underweight
18.5–24.9	Normal
25.0–29.9	Overweight
30.0–34.9	Obese
35.0–39.9	Severe obesity
≥40	Morbid obesity

5. D: The primary indications for renal replacement therapy (RRT) include fluid overload, metabolic acidosis, and hyperkalemia. Other indications include increased confusion, pericarditis, or gastrointestinal (GI) bleeding. Increasing oliguria and increasing serum creatinine require further evaluation and may trigger RRT to prevent further kidney damage. Intermittent hemodialysis (administered over 3–4 hours about three times weekly) and continuous venovenous hemofiltration are commonly used after cardiac surgery for patients requiring RRT. Continuous venovenous systems include slow continuous ultrafiltration (SCUF), continuous venovenous hemofiltration (CVVH), and continuous venovenous hemodiafiltration (CVVHD).

6. C: Retrosternal and neck pain, dyspnea, and slight neck edema indicate pneumomediastinum. Hamman's sign—a precordial rasping sound heard on auscultation during heartbeat as the heart moves against tissues filled with air—is an indication of both pneumomediastinum and

pneumopericardium but is not generally present with pneumothorax or cardiac tamponade. However, neck edema can occur with pneumomediastinum. Air leaks can occur from damage to the pleura during surgery or (less commonly) from obstructed chest tubes. Air leaks usually resolve within a few days but may require reinsertion of a chest tube.

7. B: The five phases of becoming bedridden (Zegelin, 2008) include the following:

- Phase I: Unstable gait/Imbalance, beginning difficulty with ambulation.
- Phase II: Fall or hospital stay that limits mobility because of injury or lack of assistance.
- Phase III: Prescribed bed rest and chair. Patients are often up for limited periods by choice even if ambulation is not restricted.
- Phase IV: Ability to transfer from bed to chair independently is lost. Patient is completely dependent on others.
- Phase V: 24-hour-a-day bed rest with no transfers for elimination or other needs.

8. D: Common adverse effects of calcium channel blockers, such as diltiazem or verapamil, include bradycardia, hypotension, heart failure, PR prolongation, and/or constipation. Bradycardia results from decreased sinoatrial (SA) nodal output and PR prolongations from delays in atrioventricular (AV) conduction. These drugs may cause marked hypotension and worsening of existing heart failure. Calcium channel blockers, used to treat tachycardia, block the influx of calcium ions across membranes of cardiac and arterial muscle cells, slowing the AV node conduction of impulses into the ventricles, thereby slowing the ventricular rate.

9. A: Kolb's model of experiential learning is based on acquiring knowledge through grasping experience and transforming that experience into knowledge through cognitive processes and perception. Experience may be transformed into knowledge through abstract conceptualizing (analyzing, thinking), observation of others, or actively experimenting. This model stresses that the individual makes choices between the concrete and the abstract, and this is reflected in learning styles:

- Diverging: Concrete experience and reflective observation.
- Assimilating: Abstract conceptualization and reflective observation.
- Converging: Abstract conceptualization and active experimentation.
- Accommodating: Concrete experience and reflective observation.

10. C: If a patient reports that injuries resulted from domestic violence, when documenting the abuse in the patient's health record, the AGACNP should use direct quotations to document the patient's statements. The AGACNP should make notes that are as detailed and accurate as possible, including descriptions of all injuries (size, location, extent) and any interventions because the health record may become part of a criminal proceeding.

11. D: Targeted primary prevention. Primary prevention strategies include the following:

- Targeted: Aimed at a select group or subgroup with perceived risk. Strategies may include encouraging physicians to intervene with brief advice, such as advising all adolescents about the dangers of substance abuse.
- Universal: Aimed at the entire population, nonspecific. These strategies may include mass-marketing procedures, such as multimedia antidrug campaigns aimed at the general public.
- Indicated: Aimed at individuals at high risk, such as adolescents in environments with heavy drug use.

Secondary prevention includes efforts to prevent further drug abuse, such as Narcotics Anonymous.

12. B: Monoamine oxidase inhibitors (MAOIs) should not be taken with alcohol and nonalcoholic substitutes for beer or wine, foods high in tyramine (organ meats, cured meats, caviar, cheese products, avocados, bananas, raisins, soy, and fava beans), and products containing caffeine (tea, cola, chocolate, and coffee). MAOIs are older antidepressant medications that are used less frequently now that others are available because they have significant side effects and interactions with other medications, such as decongestants, opioids, and antidepressants.

13. A: Once a person completes gender reassignment surgery and legally changes genders, that person is then considered the reassigned gender; thus, Mikaela is considered female, so her attraction to other females would result in her sexual orientation as lesbian. If she were attracted to males, she would be heterosexual. While she could also be classified as homosexual, this term is more commonly used for gay males, and she is no longer considered a male. She does not report a bisexual attraction to both genders.

14. C: Case control studies compare those with a condition (cases) to a group without (controls) to determine if the affected group has characteristics that are different. Prospective cohort studies choose a group of patients without disease, assess risk factors, and then follow the group over time to determine (prospect for) which ones develop disease. Retrospective cohort studies are initiated after a condition develops and data are collected retrospectively from medical records to evaluate whether members of the cohort selected had exposure and developed disease. Cross-sectional studies assess disease and exposure at the same time in a target population, evaluating the presence of disease at a point in time.

15. D: The patient most likely at risk is the man who shot himself in the chest while alone. A suicide risk assessment should evaluate some of the following criteria: Would the individual sign a contract for safety? Is there a suicide plan? How lethal is the plan? What is the elopement risk? How often are the suicidal thoughts, and has the person attempted suicide before? High-risk findings include the following:

- Violent suicide attempt (knives, gunshots).
- Suicide attempt with a low chance of rescue.
- Ongoing psychosis or disordered thinking.
- Ongoing severe depression and feeling of helplessness.
- History of previous suicide attempts.
- Lack of social support system.

16. B: If 15 hours after a patient was involved in an accident that resulted in a comminuted fracture of the femur the patient exhibits increasing dyspnea and tachypnea as well as confusion and difficulty speaking and a petechial rash in the mouth and upper body, the most likely cause of this triad of symptoms is fat embolism syndrome. Fat emboli enter the bloodstream and lodge in the lungs where platelets, red blood cells, and fibrin adhere to them, leading to respiratory distress syndrome. They can migrate to the skin (causing petechiae) and to the brain (causing central nervous system [CNS] problems).

17. A: Steps to conflict resolution include the following:

- First, allow both sides to present their side of conflict without bias, maintaining a focus on opinions rather than individuals.
- Encourage cooperation through negotiation and compromise.

- Maintain the focus, providing guidance to keep the discussions on track and avoid arguments.
- Evaluate the need for renegotiation, formal resolution process, or third-party involvement.

The best time for conflict resolution is when differences emerge but before open conflict and hardening of positions occur. The AGACNP must pay close attention to the people and problems involved, listen carefully, and reassure those involved that their points of view are understood.

18. B: According to the American Geriatrics Society Guideline for the Prevention of Falls in Older Persons, if a patient has one fall, the patient should be assessed for gait and balance, including the get-up-and-go test in which the patient stands up from a chair without using arms to assist, walks across the room, and returns. If the patient is steady, no further assessment is needed. If the patient demonstrates unsteadiness, further assessment to determine the cause is necessary.

19. C: With severe heart failure, ventricular remodeling (cardiac myocytes hypertrophying) may occur with the ventricle walls thinning and enlarging, resulting in a larger ventricular capacity. While the body is trying to compensate and increase cardiac output by enlarging the ventricles, the thinner walls are weaker and less able to effectively pump blood, so the ejection fraction decreases even further and the cardiac output falls. This type of pathological remodeling is not reversible.

20. D: Norovirus may remain viable on environmental surfaces, such as furniture, for up to 28 days and is resistant to freezing and high heat. For this reason, outbreaks are common and may occur in healthcare facilities, especially if hand cleaning and environmental cleaning is inadequate. Some outbreaks have been traced to infected food handlers. Twenty-five strains of Norovirus can infect humans, and Norovirus is exceptionally virulent because only 10 viral particles can cause disease.

21. B: Adolescents ages 15 to 17 should be restrained and/or secluded for no longer than 2 hours. Restraints should be used only as a last resort in cases in which the adolescent and/or others are threatened, and the patient should be released as soon as it is healthy and safe to do so. Adolescents must be frequently monitored during the use of restraints and seclusion; pressure and unsafe holds should not be applied to adolescents in restraints.

22. A: When administering platelets to a patient, the infusion should be done as fast as the patient can tolerate because platelets tend to clump together if the transfusion takes too long. Platelet concentrate is usually about 50 mL. Platelet transfusions may be given for leukemia, other malignancies, and severe thrombocytopenia. Although ABO/Rh compatibility is desired, the number of red blood cells that remain is usually too low to cause a reaction, but Rh antibodies may form if the patient is Rh−.

23. D: Frontotemporal dementia (FTD) is especially characterized by changes in personality and behavior and difficulty using and understanding language. Onset is usually between ages 40 and 45, and patients may exhibit marked personality changes, including acting inappropriately and emotional blunting. There are different variants of FTD with behavioral problems more pronounced in some and language problems (production and comprehension) in others. The only treatment is supportive. FTD may be misdiagnosed as Alzheimer's disease.

24. C: Although all of these are important, patients who are homeless require further assistance with discharge because compliance with treatment and follow-up appointments is poor in the homeless population. Interventions that are most important include the following:

- Lists of safe shelters and places they can go to bathe, eat, and get mail.
- Assistance in applying for welfare assistance or Social Security.

Discharge planning should begin on admission and must be a joint effort so that the transfer and discharge documents provide the information that the individual needs.

25. A: Drug absorption may be impaired in older adults because of decreased splanchnic (visceral) blood flow. Gastric acids tend to decrease and pH tends to become more acidic, and this, combined with decreased blood flow to the stomach, can reduce absorption. Slower gastric emptying can also affect absorption. The degree to which drug absorption may be affected can be difficult to predict, although blood levels of some drugs can be monitored.

26. D: The finding on physical assessment that is consistent with osteoarthritis is hard, nontender nodules on distal and proximal interphalangeal joints. Those on distal interphalangeal joints are called Heberden's nodes; those on proximal interphalangeal joints are called Bouchard nodes. Spindle-shaped swelling of soft tissue of proximal interphalangeal joints, ulnar deviation of the fingers, swan-neck deformity of the fingers, as well as boutonnière deformity (with the knuckle appearing as though it was pushed through a buttonhole or a keyhole) are consistent with rheumatoid arthritis.

27. B: The percutaneous endoscopic gastrostomy (PEG) tube does not have an inflatable balloon, but the tube should be stabilized by pulling gently to ensure that the internal bumper is against the abdominal wall and then sliding the external stabilizer to 1.5 cm above the skin. Replacing the PEG tube is done only if the leakage cannot be otherwise controlled. Routine skin care, including application of a barrier ointment or other skin sealant, is necessary to prevent skin breakdown. In some cases, alginates, foam dressing, gauze, or pouching may be necessary.

28. A: A positive <u>Murphy's sign</u> is indicative of cholecystitis but is negative with choledocholithiasis and ascending cholangitis. This test is not accurate for geriatric patients, so a negative finding does not rule out cholecystitis for these patients. To test for Murphy's sign, hook the fingers under the right costal margin at the midpoint, palpating deeply and ask the patient to inhale deeply. Positive results occur with pain causing the patient to stop inspiring. <u>Rovsing's sign</u>—pain in the right lower quadrant (RLQ) when left-sided abdominal pressure is applied—suggests appendicitis along with RLQ pain (rebound tenderness) on quick removal of pressure.

29. D: If a 40-year-old patient with bipolar disease has been well controlled with lithium but comes to the emergency department with influenza that has caused 2 days of severe vomiting and diarrhea, the AGACNP's priority should be to immediately obtain a lithium level. Lithium has a very narrow therapeutic range, and volume depletion resulting from nausea and/or vomiting may result in elevated serum levels, which can be life threatening. If the level drops too low (such as when the medication is vomited), then symptoms of bipolar disease may recur.

30. B: The Hamilton Anxiety Rating Scale (HAM-A) scores phrases that describe feelings and symptoms. Scores are 0 (not present), 1 (mild), 2 (moderate), 3 (severe), and 4 (incapacitating). The phrases relate to 14 issues: anxious mood, tension, fears, insomnia, intellectual, depressed mood, somatic (muscular), somatic (sensory), cardiovascular symptoms, respiratory symptoms, gastrointestinal (GI) symptoms, genitourinary (GU) symptoms, autonomic symptoms, and behavior at the interview. HAM-A assesses the psychic anxiety and the physical complaints (somatic anxiety) related to those anxieties.

31. C: A nasoenteric tube for an adult should be marked prior to insertion with measurements including the distance from nose to earlobe, plus earlobe to xiphoid process, plus 8 to 10 inches for enteric placement. Six inches are needed for gastric placement. The nasoenteric tube tip is initially placed in the stomach (verified by chest X-ray) and then moves into the small intestine through

peristalsis over about 24 hours. Proper placement should be reconfirmed before every feeding by checking the tube length measurement, aspirating and observing the aspirant, and checking pH.

32. A: Patients have a right to refuse treatment for religious or other personal reasons, so the most appropriate action is to simply provide the patient with factual information about the disease, treatments, and prognosis in a neutral manner, without trying to coerce or frighten the patient. In some cases, patients may change their minds when presented with information, but the AGACNP should remain supportive regardless of the patient's decision. Asking the family to intervene is not appropriate, and refusal of treatment alone does not suggest the need for referral to a psychologist.

33. A: If a 33-year-old female is hospitalized for treatment of acute pyelonephritis and has been receiving IV fluids and ampicillin plus aminoglycoside for the past 5 days but the patient's temperature remains elevated and she is still in pain and nauseated, the patient should likely be evaluated for perinephric abscess. With perinephric abscess, the onset of symptoms is usually slower than with other acute pyelonephritis, and fever often persists for more than 4 days.

34. D: If a patient who suffered a stroke has persistent dysphagia and cough and the AGACNP is concerned that the patient may aspirate, the most appropriate referral is to a speech pathologist. The speech pathologist is able to assess the strength of the mouth, including the lips, the tongue, the palate, and the jaw. The speech pathologist may suggest preventive measures, including positioning and diet modifications, and may prescribe exercises and/or neurological stimulation or thermostimulation.

35. B: If the AGACNP is working on a unit that has been understaffed and one of the nurses on the unit states that his blood pressure has increased because he dreads coming to work and feels that the organization doesn't value nurses or care about patients and that nothing will change, the AGACNP should recognize that the nurse is most at risk for burnout. Stages include the following:

1. Fight-or-flight response.
2. Emotional reaction: anger, shock, surprise.
3. Negative thinking.
4. Physical reaction.
5. No change in stressor or person.
6. Burnout.

36. C: If a 73-year-old patient is in the hospital with hypothermia because his daughter, who manages his finances, forgot to pay the heating bill and the heat was shut off during a cold spell, this is an example of neglect. The patient's needs were not adequately met. Neglect may be intentional or accidental. Other signs of neglect may include lack of dentures, poor nutrition, weight loss, unkempt appearance, and unsanitary living conditions. Neglect may be associated with abuse as well.

37. D: If the AGACNP is promoting evidence-based practice and using the PICOT format to pose a clinical question, the AGACNP would first focus on the patient population. PICOT is explained as follows:

PICOT format	
Patient population	What is the target population (adults, children, homeless) or setting (home care, inpatient, outpatient)?
Intervention/Area of interest	What is the potential intervention?
Comparison	What are other interventions?
Outcome	What are strategies for measuring outcomes?
Time	What is the time frame for intervention?

38. B: If a 70-year-old female with chronic obstructive pulmonary disease (COPD) has experienced an exacerbation after contracting an upper respiratory infection and her oxygen saturation level is 84%, pH is 7.29, $PaCO_2$ is 52 mm Hg, PaO_2 is 53 mm Hg, and HCO_3 is 25 mEq/L, the acid-base imbalance that the patient is experiencing is respiratory acidosis. The pH is acidotic (<7.35), the $PaCO_2$ is elevated (normal is 35 to 45 mm Hg), and the PaO_2 is at the low end of normal (normal is ≥80 mm Hg), indicating that the problem is respiratory in nature. The HCO_3 remains within normal range but near the upper limit (normal is 22 to 26 mEq/L). These findings indicate a sudden decrease in ventilation.

39. A: If the AGACNP has been asked to serve as a coach for nurses in the medical-surgical unit, then his or her initial action should be to complete a needs assessment with input from all members of the staff. The goal of coaching is to address the educational needs of the staff members, and the needs assessment will help guide the planning process and the interventions. Coaching may also include mentoring and helping to translate evidence-based research into clinical practice.

40. D: If a 27-year-old male patient has experienced increased thirst and frequency of urination, including nocturia, increased appetite but recent weight loss, and laboratory tests show glucose of 526 mg/dL (29.2 mmol/L), the urine is positive for glucose and ketones, and a blood pH of 7.22 (normal is 7.35 to 7.45), the blood pH is the result of increased ketone levels in the blood. Because insulin supply is inadequate and the glucose level is high, the body breaks down fat to use as a source of energy. As the blood lipid level increases, these lipids are metabolized, resulting in ketones as by-products, including acetoacetic acid and beta-hydroxybutyric acid. These acidic by-products increase the acidity of the blood.

41. C: A 32-year-old female reports 6 to 10 episodes of palpitation daily, irritability, insomnia, heat intolerance, eye irritation, and increased appetite coupled with weight loss. Her vital signs are BP, 170/86; P, 114; R, 20. Her temperature is 37.5°C (99.5°F), and an ECG shows atrial fibrillation. This patient should undergo thyroid function tests (T3, T4, and TSH) because these signs and symptoms are indicative of hyperthyroidism. Hyperthyroidism may be associated with Graves' disease (an autoimmune disorder), thyroiditis, or pituitary tumors.

42. A: According to Drug Enforcement Administration (DEA) regulations for schedule II drugs, no refills are allowed, although the healthcare provider may provide a patient for multiple prescriptions for the same schedule II drug to allow a 90-day supply. However, each prescription

must indicate the earliest date by which the patient can fill the prescription. Schedule II drugs include opioids and other drugs that have a high risk of abuse: cocaine, opium, morphine, methadone, Ritalin, Concerta, Focalin, oxycodone, oxymorphone, fentanyl, hydromorphone, hydrocodone (pure), codeine (=/> 90 mg per unit dose), secobarbital, meperidine, pentobarbital, and amphetamine.

43. C: Although asthma attacks and chronic obstructive pulmonary disease (COPD) exacerbations may be difficult to distinguish based on X-rays, signs and symptoms, and laboratory tests, some characteristics can help to distinguish the two:

- Onset of asthma is at a younger age (usually <30) than COPD, which most often occurs after age 40.
- Asthma attacks can usually be fairly quickly resolved with treatment, but COPD responds more slowly and often only temporarily.
- Asthma has a genetic component, but COPD generally does not.
- Asthma patients are much less likely to have been smokers, whereas almost all COPD patients have smoked.

44. D: If a patient with a T-6 spinal cord injury is lying flat in bed but suddenly exhibits blurred vision, severe headache, piloerection with flushing above the lesion and pallor below, and markedly elevated BP of 280/160, the first action should be to elevate the head of the bed to 45°. Then the patient's bladder should be checked for distension or the catheter checked for kinks and distension relieved, clothes loosened, and bowels checked. If symptoms continue after the stimulus is identified and relieved, the patient may need an alpha-adrenergic blocker or vasodilator, such as nifedipine.

45. B: The teaching strategy that is the most efficient approach for a group of 8 patients regarding the need for lifestyle changes needed to manage hypertension and heart disease is lecture-discussion. This format allows the AGACNP to provide information in a short-lecture format and then provides the patients time to ask questions and discuss the information shared. Supplemental printed materials may be provided to the patients. The AGACNP should cover no more than 5 to 7 different topics in one session.

46. A: The "talk and die" phenomenon in which a patient loses consciousness after a blow to the head and then recovers and appears to be fine before suddenly developing severe symptoms of brain injury is typical of epidural hemorrhage, which is bleeding between the skull and the dura mater, resulting in compression of the underlying brain tissue. With rapid treatment, prognosis is good, but if the lesion expands rapidly, a midline shift and herniation may occur.

47. C: If, when conducting a history and physical exam of a patient with dyspnea, the AGACNP discovers that the patient has smoked two packs (40 cigarettes) daily for at least 15 years, this represents 30 pack-years. One pack-year is equal to smoking one pack (20) of cigarettes daily for a year. The greater the number of pack-years, the higher the risk of developing COPD. Most patients with COPD have smoked for 40 pack-years, and symptoms are not usually evident until more than 20 pack-years of smoking.

48. D: If a nonverbal patient with dementia is frowning and grimacing on movement, crying out periodically, and lying rigid or in the fetal position, the AGACNP should recognize that the patient is likely in pain. Pain Assessment in Advanced Dementia (PAINAD) is a tool to help evaluate signs of pain in those with dementia through observation of respirations (increased labored), vocalizations

(moaning, groaning), facial expressions (frown, grimace, sad), body language (tense, fidgeting, rigid, fetal position), and consolability.

49. B: If a 60-year-old African-American patient has a body mass index (BMI) of 32 kg/m², hemoglobin A1C level of 7.1 (71 mmol/L), fasting serum glucose level of 152 mg/dL (8.4mmol/L), triglyceride level of 168, and high-density lipoprotein (HDL) level of 24 mg/dL, and the patient is diagnosed with insulin resistance and diabetes mellitus, type 2, the drug of choice for initiating therapy is usually a biguanide, typically metformin. Metformin is usually tolerated well and does not cause hypoglycemia. If the A1C levels haven't fallen to below 7% within about 3 months, then an additional medication is prescribed.

50. A: Following lunch, if a 72-year-old female experiences a sudden episode of loss of vision in the right eye during which the patient feels dizzy and weak, and her speech is slightly garbled but the symptoms clear within 15 to 20 minutes, the most likely diagnosis is transient ischemic episode (TIE). Transient impaired vision of one eye (amaurosis fugax) is a common finding with TIE, which is often a precursor to a stroke, so the patient should undergo a complete examination.

51. C: The method of wound debridement that should generally be avoided is wet-to-dry dressings. Although this method of debridement was in common use for many years, it actually disrupts granulation and is no longer recommended. Various other methods of debridement, such as irrigation, chemical debridement (enzyme debriding agents), hydrotherapy (used commonly for burns), and sharp debridement, may be used depending on the extent of the wound and the presence of slough and eschar.

52. A: If the medical-surgical unit has experienced an outbreak of *Clostridium difficile* infections involving 10 patients over a 2-week period, in order to reduce the transmission of the infection, the AGACNP is working with staff members and should concentrate efforts on the use of proper contact precautions and hand hygiene because the infection is easily spread by contaminated hands. The spores can remain viable on environmental surfaces for long periods of time. Housekeeping procedures should also be reviewed.

53. D: If a 16-year-old comes to the emergency department with a sore reddened and blistering area on his left lower leg and the patient states he believes he was bitten by a spider but didn't actually see the spider, the AGACNP should suspect that the patient may have a *Staphylococcus aureus* infection. Staph infections are frequently mistaken for spider bites and should always be considered when the spider is not observed. Additionally, many types of spider bites are not poisonous and do not cause severe reactions.

54. B: If a patient with heart failure has developed pulmonary edema and has rales and rhonchi present throughout the lung fields, is very anxious, and the initial treatment includes 15 L oxygen per nonrebreather mask, furosemide 60 mg IV, nitroglycerine, nitroprusside, and morphine to reduce anxiety, the initial goal of therapy should be to maintain the PaO_2 at greater than 60 mm Hg. Although the normal PaO_2 ranges from 80 to 95 mm Hg, the critical value is less than 45 mm Hg, at which point perfusion is inadequate.

55. A: If a patient is taking atorvastatin for dyslipidemia, a bile acid sequestrant may be recommended for its additive effect to reduce the risk of cardiac mortality resulting from dyslipidemia. Bile acid sequestrants are resins that bind bile acids and prevent reabsorption and are effective in lowering low-density lipoprotein (LDL) cholesterol. They are sometimes used along with statins, whereas fibrates should be avoided because combining them with statins may result in an increased risk of rhabdomyolysis.

56. D: If a patient has suspected heart failure, B-type natriuretic peptide (BNP) is the laboratory test that will show the severity of heart failure. This hormone is secreted by ventricular tissues in response to increased volume and pressure in the ventricles, as occurs with heart failure. Normal values should be less than 100 pg/mL (100 ng/mL). A level of 250 pg/mL (250 ng/L) is consistent with mild heart failure, 375 pg/mL (375 ng/L) with moderate, 650 pg/mL (650 ng/L) with moderately severe, and 800 pg/mL (800 ng/L) with severe.

57. C: If the AGACNP is using the beliefs, values, meanings, goals, and relationships (BVMGR) rubric for implementing spiritual care, these aspects apply to assessment of the patient. That is, the AGACNP should try to understand the patient's BVMGR and should not let personal BVMGR intrude and should avoid any indication of proselytizing when the AGACNP's BVMGR is at odds with the patient. Although the AGACNP may not share the patient's belief system, the AGACNP should always seek to understand and to show respect for it.

58. B: If a patient with pulmonary arterial hypertension (World Health Organization disease type II [WHO II]) has started treatment with combination therapy that initially includes ambrisentan 5 mg (Letairis) and tadalafil 20 mg (Adcirca) as well as supplementary oxygen for exertion, when educating the patient about disease management, the AGACNP should tell the patient to be especially alert for signs of peripheral edema, the most common adverse effect. In some cases, pulmonary edema may also occur. Diuretic therapy, such as furosemide, may be added to the regimen. The patient should also have hemoglobin levels monitored routinely because of the increased risk of anemia.

59. A: If a patient with inflammatory bowel disease (IBD) has bouts of severe diarrhea but is unsure of the cause, the AGACNP should advise the patient to maintain a food diary, writing down all food and fluid intake to see if a pattern emerges. Although many patients with IBD are lactose intolerant, testing can show if this is the problem. Increasing fat or fiber in the diet may aggravate the diarrhea.

60. C: If an alert 70-year-old female patient hospitalized with a vertebral fracture and no previous history of incontinence has started having both urinary and fecal leakage, the AGACNP's initial response should be to examine the patient for a fecal impaction. Fecal impaction is a common cause of both urinary and fecal incontinence in patients who are hospitalized or immobile, especially if they are receiving opioids.

61. B: If a patient with latex allergy is inadvertently exposed to latex and develops severe anaphylaxis with difficulty breathing, the priority intervention is to establish an airway and administer epinephrine. The epinephrine should be administered intramuscularly into the vastus lateralis (thigh) muscle instead of the deltoid because absorption is more rapid. Patients should receive adjunctive therapy with an antihistamine (such as diphenhydramine), corticosteroid (to prevent a biphasic reaction), and an H_2 blocker (such as ranitidine).

62. D: Absorption of nutrients from the small bowel is often impaired in older adults because of broadening and shortening of villi, which decreases the surface area available. Additionally, levels of some enzymes decrease. For example, lactase levels may fall, and this can cause increased lactose intolerance. When fecal material moves slowly through the bowels, bacterial overgrowth may occur, and this can affect the absorption of nutrients because the bacteria require nutrients and can also cause diarrhea, which interferes with absorption.

63. A: A 22-year-old patient who is on a strict vegan diet is most at risk for vitamin B_{12} deficiency because vitamin B_{12} is found in animal products. Signs and symptoms include glossitis because of changes in mucosal cells, anorexia, diarrhea, and low hemoglobin with leukopenia and

thrombocytopenia. The nervous system is impaired, beginning with the peripheral nerves and paresthesias and progressing to problems with balance and proprioception. Dementia may occur.

64. B: If the AGACNP needs to delegate a task to a licensed vocational or practical nurse (LVN/LPN) but is unsure how the nurse performs because the AGACNP has not worked with this LVN/LPN before, the best initial approach is to ask the LVN/LPN how he or she would go about doing the task. Then, the AGACNP should share expectations and any specific instructions, including under what conditions and when the LVN/LPN needs to report to the AGACNP and how the AGACNP will supervise.

65. C: The AGACNP should recommend the herpes zoster (shingles) vaccine (Zostavax) for adults age 60 and older. The vaccine decreases the incidence of shingles by 51% and the incidence of postherpetic neuralgia by 67%. People who have already had shingles may still benefit from the vaccination because shingles can recur. Adults born prior to 1980 are considered immune to varicella even if they don't recall having the disease and do not need the varicella vaccination, only the herpes zoster. Contraindications include allergy to gelatin, neomycin, or other components of the vaccination, pregnancy, and immunocompromised patients.

66. B: If the AGACNP notes that one nursing team member often avoids taking care of older patients and sometimes makes disparaging remarks about the elderly, the most appropriate response is for the AGACNP to discuss attitudes toward aging with the nurse. People who exhibit ageism are often concerned about their own aging and may be unaware of their bias against older adults. However, the AGACNP should also make clear that older patients must receive the same quality of care as younger patients and that negative comments about the elderly are inappropriate.

67. D: Acute kidney injury may occur with sepsis because of decreased renal perfusion and is a common cause of acute kidney injury in patients who are critically ill, occurring in about 20% of patients with mild to moderate sepsis but in more than 50% of those with septic shock. With acute kidney injury, the patient may have a sudden increase in blood urea nitrogen (BUN) and/or serum creatinine levels and may experience oliguria. Symptoms are often associated with uremia and include nausea, vomiting, malaise, and altered sensorium. Hypertension may occur.

68. A: If a patient with fulminant hepatic failure is not a candidate for liver transplant and has signs of increasing intracranial pressure, the AGACNP should advise member of the care team to elevate the head of the bed to 30° and pad the side rails. The patient is at risk for possible seizures and must be monitored carefully with frequent neurological examinations. The patient should be maintained in a quiet environment without excess stimulation, but sedatives, which may increase drowsiness and fail to adequate metabolize, should be avoided.

69. C: Patients typically begin experiencing blackouts at a blood alcohol level of 0.20 g/100 mL. At this level, patients are severely drunk, confused, and disoriented and may have difficulty standing or walking. Patients may experience nausea and vomiting and are at increased risk of aspiration because of impaired gag reflex. Although state laws vary, persons with blood alcohol levels of 0.07 to 0.9 are considered legally drunk with impaired judgment and self-control. Patients often believe they are less impaired than they actually are.

70. D: In order to optimize venous return and prevent pressure areas for a patient who is bedridden or has limited activity, as much as possible, the head of the patient's bed should be maintained at 30° or lower. Other measures include turning patients every 2 hours, avoiding friction and shear, using positioning devices, shifting weight for chair-bound patients every 15 minutes, managing

incontinence and keeping skin clean and dry, using pressure-relief devices/mattresses, and ensuring adequate fluid and nutrition.

71. B: If an 80-year-old patient with a history of intra-abdominal surgery and diverticulosis has a simple incomplete small-bowel obstruction (without compromised blood flow) and has had nausea and vomiting for 2 days, the initial interventions that are most indicated are nasogastric (NG) decompression and IV fluids (isotonic). The patient will likely also require potassium replacement because hypokalemia is commonly associated with bowel obstruction and vomiting. The most likely cause (and the most common) for small-bowel obstruction is adhesions.

72. A: If an 18-year-old patient became angry at her parents and ingested 10,000 mg of extra-strength acetaminophen and was found by her parents 12 hours later, pale, nauseated, and diaphoretic but without vomiting, the AGACNP should recognize that the patient is at risk for liver failure. The maximum dose for acetaminophen in 24 hours is 4000 mg, and severe liver damage can occur at 7000 mg. The chance for recovery is good if treatment is instituted within 8 hours of ingestion.

73. A: If the AGACNP is newly hired at a healthcare organization and believes that there is a need for improvement in patient care, the first thing that the AGACNP should assess is the workplace culture. The AGACNP should determine which members of the staff have the most influence over decisions and should determine the values, attitudes, and beliefs of the organization and staff and the degree to which the culture is receptive to change. Immediately proposing changes without first understanding the workplace culture may lead to discord and resistance.

74. C: If the AGACNP notes that a patient's blood pressure has fallen precipitously and the pulse rate has increased but fails to take action and the patient suffers permanent injury as a result, the element of malpractice that applies to the AGACNP is breach of duty owed. Duty owed to the patient is usually established by employment records or agreements to provide care, and breach of duty owed to the patient occurs when a nurse who has a duty to care for a patient provides care that is below standards.

75. B: If a patient with ptosis and extraocular weakness with a presumed diagnosis of myasthenia gravis is undergoing the Tensilon (edrophonium chloride) challenge and has a positive finding, the symptoms (ptosis and extraocular weakness) should improve. Tensilon (which prevents acetylcholine from breaking down) is administered by IV and then the patient is observed for improvement and asked to carry out a number of activities, such as sitting and standing, holding arms up until they tire, and counting backward until the voice tires.

76. B: Because of some risk of ABO incompatibility, administration of type O packed red blood cells to a patient who comes to the emergency department vomiting bright-red blood and is hemodynamically unstable is usually withheld until typing and cross-matching is completed. However, volume resuscitation should immediately be carried out with 0.9% saline or lactated Ringer's solution while waiting for the results. A nasogastric tube is usually not necessary, and gastric lavage is contraindicated.

77. C: If the AGACNP has instituted staff rounding with the goal of meeting with each staff member at least once weekly, the purpose of staff rounding is to improve communication and support staff members' needs. Typical questions include asking about what's working well, who should be recognized for good work, what needs to be improved, whether the staff member has the needed tools and equipment, and whether the person needs help. The overall goal is to improve staff satisfaction and reduce turnover.

78. C: If the AGACNP has taught a patient's spouse to change the patient's dressing and to understand signs of healing and infection, the best method to ensure that the patient's spouse is able to carry out the dressing change and monitor the wound is to ask for a return demonstration. The AGACNP should ask the spouse to change the dressing while the AGACNP observes and to "talk through" the steps during the procedure, including a description of the wound.

79. A: If a patient has acute nongonococcal bacterial (septic) arthritis of the knee, the immediate treatment includes antibiotics and drainage of the joint. Treatment is initiated with broad-spectrum antibiotics until culture and sensitivity returns. Drainage of the joint usually includes arthroscopic lavage and debridement with a drain placed into the joint. Symptoms are usually acute with pain, swelling, and heat in the joint as well as fever and chills. Patients should begin early active range-of-motion (ROM) exercises to tolerance.

80. B:. If a 32-year-old patient suffered carbon monoxide (CO) toxicity and is receiving 100% oxygen per nonrebreather mask, the patient should be maintained on 100% oxygen therapy until he or she is asymptomatic and the hemoglobin CO level falls to less than 10%. If the initial level was greater than 15%, the patient should be evaluated for cardiovascular complications. Pregnant patients with levels greater than 15% and other patients with a level of greater than 40% should be referred for hyperbaric treatment.

81. D: If a 73-year-old patient has a 6 cm by 4 cm coccygeal pressure ulcer coccygeal ulcer that extends to the muscle and is partially covered with black necrotic tissue, the AGACNP would classify the pressure ulcer as stage IV. The National Pressure Ulcer Advisory Panel (NPUAP) stages are classified as follows:

NPUAP pressure ulcer classification	
Suspected	Blood blister, discolored skin, pain, texture change, or temperature change.
Stage I	Localized nonblanching reddened area.
Stage II	Partial-thickness skin loss involving epidermis and dermis. Abrasion/Blistered appearance.
Stage III	Exposure of subcutaneous tissue, but not of muscle or bone.
Stage IV	Extends to muscle, bone, tendons, or joints with extensive damage and necrosis.
Unstageable	Slough and/or eschar in wound makes staging impossible until debridement.

82. A: If the AGACNP intends to implement a new procedure in the delivery of patient care, the AGACNP should understand that the biggest threat to implementation of change is usually staff resistance. For this reason, it's important for the AGACNP to obtain "buy in" as part of preparation and to identify and recruit key individuals who are likely to influence others to promote change. Staff resistance can be passive (lack of enthusiasm, complaining) or active (refusing to participate, undermining efforts).

83. B: If the AGACNP overhears another nurse complaining that an adult female Hmong patient is subservient and dependent because she allows her father to make decisions about her health care and that the nurse tried without success to convince the patient to make her own decisions, this type of intervention would best be described as cultural imposition. The nurse is trying to impose a cultural norm that is different from that of the patient. In the Hmong community, the eldest male in the family is usually the one to make decisions, and this is a respected tradition.

84. A: If a 21-year-old African-American female presents with a malar rash, Raynaud's phenomenon, joint pain and stiffness, positive antinuclear antibody (ANAs), and thrombocytopenia of 90,000/mcL, the probable diagnosis is systemic lupus erythematosus (SLE), which is an inflammatory autoimmune disorder. About 85% of cases occur in females, and African-Americans have a rate about 4 times higher than Caucasians. The malar "butterfly" rash occurs in fewer than 50% of patients, but other cutaneous manifestations, such as splinter hemorrhages, may be present.

85. A: When the AGACNP is assessing a patient with neurological injury, an <u>upper motor neuron lesion</u> is indicated by muscle spasticity. Other indications include hyperactive reflexes, loss of voluntary muscle control, and increased muscle tone but no evidence of muscle atrophy. However, with a <u>lower motor neuron lesion</u>, although the patient also lacks voluntary muscle control, he or she exhibits decreased muscle tone and muscle flaccidity as well as decreased or absent reflexes and atrophy of muscles.

86. D: If a 66-year-old patient with a history of alcoholic cirrhosis has developed small esophageal varices but no bleeding, the most appropriate preventive treatment is a nonselective beta-blocker, such as propranolol. The goal of this treatment is to reduce the hepatic venous pressure gradient to less than 12 mm Hg because higher pressure increases the risk of bleeding. Endoscopic band ligation is as effective in preventing bleeding as nonselective beta-blockers but poses more risks of complications so is usually reserved as a second-line treatment.

87. B: If a 25-year-old patient's body mass index (BMI) is 17.5 (normal is 18.5 to 24.9), the patient is underweight and likely lacks adequate caloric intake. The patient's albumin level is within normal limits at 3.8 g/dL (38 g/L), reflecting adequate long-term protein intake; however, the prealbumin level is low at 6 mg/dL (60 mg/L) (normal is 16 to 40 mg/dL *or* 160 to 400 mg/L). Prealbumin has a half-life of 2 to 3 days (compared to 18 to 20 for albumin), so the findings reflect acute (short-term) protein malnutrition.

88. C: If the AGACNP has proposed use of the Situation-Background-Assessment-Recommendation (SBAR) format for hand-off communication but is encountering resistance from long-time staff members who dislike change, the best method of dealing with resistance is to encourage staff members to express opinions and discuss concerns. The AGACNP should answer any questions, provide evidence of benefits, and respond to misperceptions. When change is evidence-based and in the best interests of the patients, leadership may require change without voting.

89. A: If the AGACNP hears a patient's physician complaining that a patient is "difficult and impatient," and the AGACNP tells the physician that the patient is very frightened and acting defensively, the aspect of care that the nurse is exhibiting is advocacy. The AGACNP is speaking up in defense of the patient and acting for the patient's benefit in trying to help the physician have a more balanced view of the patient's behavior.

90. A: In the event of a disaster, increasing surge capacity allows for admission of a large number of injured clients. The initial strategy is to identify clients safely eligible for early discharge. This may also include canceling scheduled procedures, such as elective surgeries. Extra beds can be placed in outpatient areas and in hallways because this is more time-effective than attempting to transfer existing patients to different rooms and cleaning and preparing the rooms. In some cases, non-disaster-related clients may be diverted to other hospitals; but in most cases, other facilities will also be impacted by the disaster.

91. D: Paroxetine hydrochloride 20 mg P.O. daily in AM is a correct representation of an order in an electronic health record (EHR) with a medication order set. Large doses (in the millions) should be

ordered in words, "6 million units" rather than 6,000,000, and the word "units" should be spelled out. Order sets should not use abbreviations for medications, such as "ASA" for aspirin. Micrograms should be abbreviated as mcg rather than µg, and the medication dosage should not precede the name of the medication.

92. A: When confidential patient data are contained on mobile devices, such as smartphones or personal digital assistants (PDAs), these devices should contain locking and tracking software so that the data cannot be accessed and the device can be located. Some software is also available that allows distance deletion of data if the device is misplaced or stolen. The organization should have clear policies in place for handling the loss of mobile devices or misuse in order to protect patient confidentiality.

93. C: If a patient has been diagnosed with tuberculosis (TB), the first-line drug susceptibility testing (liquid medium) takes 1 to 2 weeks before results are available. This test should routinely be carried out on the original isolate to ensure that the medication selected is effective. The goal of treatment is to destroy all tubercle bacilli and prevent the emergence of clinically significant drug resistance. Patients must be well educated about the importance of adherence because nonadherence is a primary cause of treatment failure, transmission of TB, and drug resistance.

94. B: The Joint Commission requires two identifiers to ensure that the correct individual is receiving care and that the care is intended for that individual. Identifiers must be specific to the patient. The first identifier is usually the patient's name, often found on the wristband, and the second can be the birthdate, patient ID number, or telephone number. Birthplace is usually too nonspecific as is place of employment. If an armband is used as an identifier, it must be on the patient's body and cannot be simply placed at the bedside or taped to a bedside stand.

95. B: Bundling occurs when an insurance plan negotiates a specific fee for a procedure, including all associated costs, and pays one bill. Unbundling occurs when a bundled agreement is dissolved, and the insurance plan pays separate bills (hospital, anesthesiologist, surgeon, etc.). Fee-for-service is the traditional billing method in which services are billed for separately. Discounted fee-for-service is similar to fee-for-service except that reimbursements are discounted.

96. D: If a 25-year-old patient has developed itchy, red, sharply defined, scaly lesions in both axillae, the additional finding that supports a diagnosis of psoriasis is fine stippling of the fingernails. Some drugs (beta-blockers antimalarials, statins, and lithium) may worsen or trigger a flare-up. Patients should avoid corticosteroids because severe rebound flare-ups can occur when the drug is tapered. Psoriasis should be managed by a dermatologist with experience treating it.

97. A: Nurse practitioners (NPs) may bill Medicare for services in accordance with state restrictions and supervision requirements. The NP must bill using a National Provider Identification (NPI) number and meet the educational and licensing requirements for NPs. Some states require direct supervision by a physician on the premises, whereas others require indirect or periodical supervision. The Centers for Medicare and Medicaid Services (CMS) pay for NP services that are medically necessary, equivalent to physician services, accurately documented on medical records, and billed correctly. Medicare may directly reimburse the NP if state law allows.

98. C: According to Knowles, adult learners tend to be practical and goal-oriented, so they like to remain organized and keep their goal in mind while learning. Other characteristics of adult learners include the following:

- Self-directed: Adults like active involvement and responsibility.
- Knowledgeable: Adults can relate new material to information with which they are familiar by life experience or education.
- Relevancy-oriented: Adults like to know how they will use information.
- Motivated: Adults like to see evidence of their own achievement, such as by gaining a certificate.

99. B: The ethnic group that has the highest prevalence of asthma is African-American, especially among children, with the rate in African-American children almost 60% higher than in Caucasian children. Rates are also high among Native Americans and those of Puerto Rican descent. Because of the disparity in rates of asthma, children in these ethnic groups should be routinely screened for signs of asthma, preventive treatment should be prescribed as indicated, and parents/caregivers should be educated about environmental triggers.

100. B: Healthcare Common Procedure Coding System (HCPCS) level II E codes are used when filing a Medicare claim for durable medical equipment, such as a bedside commode. D codes are used for dental procedures and include the Current Dental Terminology (CDT) code set copyrighted by the American Dental Association (ADA). L codes are used for orthotic and prosthetic procedures and devices such as orthopedic shoes. P codes are used for pathology and laboratory services.

101. D: If, one week after a tick bite, a patient develops erythema migrans (15 cm diameter) (a bull's-eye rash) with slight burning at the bite site, in an area endemic to Lyme disease, the treatment of choice is doxycycline 100 mg BID for 2 to 3 weeks. Lyme disease is caused by the spirochete *Borrelia burgdorferi*. Although some patients are asymptomatic, Lyme disease can cause flu-like symptoms, joint pain, arthritis, and severe neurological disorders.

102. C: The Health Insurance Portability and Accountability Act of 1996 (HIPAA) Security Rule applies to protected health information (PHI) that is transmitted electronically. The Security Rule was developed to meet the requirements of the HIPAA Privacy Rule. The Security Rule requires that safeguards (administrative, physical, and technical) be in place to protect electronic health information from threats, hazards, and nonpermitted disclosures. Access must be limited to authorized users only. Other safeguards include automatic logoff and encryption and decryption of protected healthcare information.

103. A: Tinnitus and low-frequency hearing loss are typically present with vertigo associated with Ménière's syndrome (endolymphatic hydrops) and help to differentiate it from vertigo associated with migraines, which are more often associated with headache, photosensitivity, and head pressure. Typically, patients with Ménière's syndrome have episodes of vertigo that last from 20 minutes to several hours. In addition to tinnitus and fluctuating low-frequency hearing loss, patients may feel pressure in the inner ear.

104. C: Health literacy is directly affected by general literacy, so when educating patients, the AGACNP should realize that the approximate percentage of adults in the U.S. who are classified as illiterate or low literate is 50%. More than 20% of the population is classified as functionally illiterate, and between 25% and 30% is low literate. Printed education materials for these patients should include illustrations and pictures with minimal text written at about the 4th-grade level.

105. B: If a 72-year-old patient has polyps removed, the type of polyp that is precancerous is the adenomatous polyp, which can include tubular adenomas, tubulovillous adenoma, and villous adenoma. Polyps associated with hereditary polyposis syndromes (familial adenomatous polyposis) are also precancerous. Patients with precancerous polyps are generally advised to have routine follow-up colonoscopies every 3 years because of the increased risk of colon cancer.

106. C: Female patients should generally be advised to begin breast cancer screening with routine mammograms at about age 40 to 50. The breast tissue is denser in younger women, so the mammogram results are less accurate. Although authorities differ in the frequency with which mammograms should be done and the starting age, most recommend that female patients have mammograms every one to two years. Although some authorities recommend screening beginning at age 40, the American Cancer Society recommends beginning at age 45 and the U.S. Preventive Services Task Force at age 50.

107. D: The condition that may pose the greatest risk for the development of breast cancer is atypical ductal hyperplasia. Hyperplasia, an overgrowth of tissue, within the ducts or lobes of the breast increases the risk up to 5 times if atypical. Ductal hyperplasia without atypia doubles the risk. If a woman has hyperplasia and a family history of breast cancer, the risk increases as well. Benign lesions that are not associated with overgrowth of breast tissue (such as lipoma and hemangioma) do not increase a person's risk.

108. A: An adolescent younger than 18 can access or refuse emergency contraception without parental knowledge or consent across the United States. Although the product information states the contraception is intended for those 17 and older, in fact, no ID is required to purchase emergency contraception, so it is available to younger adolescents. In most states, abortions for adolescents require parental knowledge or consent of some kind (one parent, both parents). Chemotherapy and transfusions require parental consent, although the adolescent's opinion may be considered.

109. B: If the AGACNP has prescribed acetaminophen for a 78-year-old patient, the AGACNP should advise the patient to limit total dosage to 2 g in 24 hours because older adults may not metabolize the drug as effectively as younger adults (who may have a total dosage of 3 to 4 g in 24 hours). Those of any age with liver disease must not exceed 2 g daily, and if the liver damage is severe, he or she should avoid acetaminophen altogether.

110. A: 4, 2, 1, and 3. The highest priority is the infected ingrown toenail because of the high risk of amputation with diabetes and foot injuries or infections. The second highest priority is diabetes mellitus, type 2, because the A1C of 8% indicates that control is poor, and this could cause the increase in blood pressure, which should be attended to next. Neuropathy of both feet is a chronic condition, also likely worsened by the diabetes mellitus, and it has the lowest priority.

111. C: The AGACNP is educating a patient who is to be discharged after surgery to remove a cancerous lesion of the colon and create a colostomy. The AGACNP advises the patient that some foods may cause:

- Odor: fish, eggs, onions, broccoli, asparagus, and cabbage.
- Gas: beans, carbonated beverages, strong cheeses, beer, and sprouts.
- Diarrhea: beer, green beans, coffee, raw fruits, spicy foods, and spinach.
- Obstruction: popcorn, seeds, raw vegetables, nuts, and corn.

112. A: If an Orthodox Jewish male patient needs an examination, and the AGACNP is female, the nurse should ask the patient if he would prefer to be examined by a male nurse. Many Orthodox Jewish males feel very uncomfortable being touched by a female and may refuse. If no male nurse is available, the patient should be advised. In that case, if the physician is male, then the part of the examination that involves touching the person may be done by the physician.

113. D: When collecting a medication history, the AGACNP should include prescription drugs, over-the-counter (OTC) drugs, vitamins, and any other health-related substances, including those that are topical or inhaled. Patients may take herbal or homeopathic substances and neglect to include them, but they can, in some instances, affect the absorption of other prescribed medications. Patients often to forget to include vitamin supplements unless asked specifically about them.

114. B: Benzodiazepines (alprazolam, diazepam, lorazepam, and chlordiazepoxide) are antianxiety drugs that should be avoided in frail elderly adults because these drugs can increase the risk of falls. Most adverse effects are associated with depression of the central nervous system (CNS) and include headache, lethargy, hypotension, and dizziness. Benzodiazepines should not be taken with alcohol or tobacco. Some other drugs may increase CNS depression, including cimetidine, disulfiram, and monoamine oxidase inhibitors (MAOIs). Some patients may have paradoxical reactions to benzodiazepines and develop hyperactive responses.

115. C: If a patient who appears to be a drug seeker demands a prescription for OxyContin for severe chronic migraine headaches, the best response is likely to verify the patient's medical history with previous healthcare providers. If the patient is unwilling to provide this information or if the information provided is incorrect, these are further indications of drug-seeking behavior. The patient should be thoroughly examined, and the extent of the examination and the questions asked should be documented.

116. B: If a patient telephones an ambulatory care center with complaints of abdominal pain and the AGACNP is screening the patient, the additional symptoms that should result in the nurse advising the patient to hang up and call 9-1-1 are increasing shortness of breath and chest discomfort because these may suggest severe cardiovascular problems, such as a myocardial infarction or aortic aneurysm. The patient should be advised to be seen in the office as soon as possible with mild fever or with mild nausea and vomiting. Patients with severe constipation should usually be seen within 24 to 48 hours.

117. A: If a 22-year-old female patient who is nulliparous and sexually active with multiple sex partners presents in the emergency department with chills and a temperature of 39°C, purulent vaginal discharge, lower abdominal pain, and cervical and adnexal tenderness, and ectopic pregnancy is ruled out, the patient should receive treatment for probable pelvic inflammatory disease with immediate antibiotics. If possible, the patient's sexual partners should also be identified and treated.

118. D: The hematology test that is outside of normal parameters for an adult male is a white blood cell (WBC) count of 4100/mm³. Normal values range from about 4500 to 11,000/mm³. A normal red blood cell (RBC) count is 4.5 to 6 million/mm³ for males and 4.0 to 5.5 million/mm³ for females. Normal hemoglobin ranges from 13 to 18 g/dL for males and 12 to 16 g/dL for females. Normal hematocrit ranges from 42% to 52% for males and from 36% to 45% for females.

119. D: Tremors and jerking movements are consistent with opioid-induced myoclonus, which may be caused by a range of drugs, including opioids and quinolones. In this case, changing to an equianalgesic should relieve symptoms in one to two days. If the myoclonus is very mild, a

benzodiazepine at bedtime may keep jerking from awakening the patient. Although similar symptoms may occur with brain metastasis, it is an uncommon metastasis with prostate cancer. Anxiety may also produce similar symptoms, but they should be less pronounced and less likely to cause jerking during sleep. Damage to the spine would produce different symptoms.

120. C: The AGACNP should remain supportive and nonjudgmental. "I'll stay with him, and you can come and go as you feel comfortable" supports the daughter's stated desire while still leaving open the opportunity for her to spend time with her father during the death vigil. People react in very different ways to death, and many people have never seen a deceased person and may be very frightened. While some people find comfort in being with a dying friend or family member, this should never be imposed on anyone.

121. B: These symptoms are consistent with obstruction of the small intestines. Sudden and frequent nausea and vomiting in large volumes, often immediately after intake, usually indicates that a bowel obstruction is in the small intestines, whereas obstructions of the colon usually result in more delayed vomiting, with fecal emesis. If obstruction is partial or inoperable, dexamethasone may relieve some of the symptoms because it reduces inflammation and swelling as well as providing relief of nausea.

122: A: If a 32-year-old male presents with swelling, erythema, and severe pain of the metatarsophalangeal (MTP) joint of the right great toe after a night of excessive drinking, and lab testing shows elevated uric acid, confirming an acute gout attack, the most appropriate treatment is a nonsteroidal anti-inflammatory drug (NSAID), such as indomethacin or ibuprofen. Colchicine should not be used to treat acute flare-ups. Corticosteroids should be reserved for those intolerant of NSAIDs. Antibiotics are not indicated because this is not an infective process.

123. B: Lymphedema: Hard, nonpitting edema with skin thickening but no pigmentation. Edema usually includes feet and toes and often occurs bilaterally. Orthostatic edema: Occurs with prolonged sitting and is soft and pitting but without skin thickening or pigmentation. It is always bilateral and includes edema of the foot. Lipedema: Bilateral fatty deposition in legs may mimic edema, but there is no pitting, skin thickening, or pigmentation and no edema of the foot. Chronic venous insufficiency: Edema is soft and pitting initially but may harden later. Skin thickening may occur around the ankle, and pigmentation changes are common. Edema often involves feet and is sometimes bilateral.

124. C: Undermining, which is damaged tissue under intact skin, usually occurs around the perimeter of a wound. Undermining is reported in centimeters and in relation to the open wound by reference to a clock face: "Extends 1.8 cm width from 1 o'clock to 4 o'clock." If the undermining is open, it can be measured by insertion of a sterile swab. In some cases, tissue may be damaged but it remains intact; in that case, undermining is estimated by palpation because undermined tissue may feel spongy.

125. B: If, while conducting a peer review, the AGACNP observes the other nurse using nontherapeutic communication techniques with a patient, the best response is to discuss the observations at a post-review meeting because the nurse is not being negligent, so there is no need to intervene immediately or report the observation. During the discussion, the AGACNP should prompt the other nurse by stating, "How did you feel about your communication with the patient?"

126. C: The four nonverbal behaviors associated with active listening include the following:

- Sit across from the patient: Facing the patient directly helps to convey interest.
- Maintain open posture: Keeping the arms and legs uncrossed helps to show that the person is open to the other person's ideas and is less defensive than a closed position.
- Lean forward: Leaning toward the patient slightly shows engagement in the interaction.
- Maintain eye contact: Maintaining eye contact helps to show interest in the person; however, the AGACNP should keep cultural differences in mind because direct eye contact is not the norm in all cultures

127. A: If a 20-year-old patient with Tourette's syndrome has increasing social problems and academic problems, often having difficulty completing activities, the common comorbidity for which the patient should be evaluated is obsessive-compulsive disorder (OCD). Between 30% and 50% of patients with Tourette's develop OCD, and up to 80% exhibit obsessive behavior. Adults with Tourette's and OCD are at risk for attention-deficit/hyperactivity disorder (ADHD) and self-injurious behavior, such as picking at scabs, self-cutting, head banging, and self-burning.

128. D: If a 16-year-old patient identifying as a girl is found to be genetically male with complete androgen insensitivity syndrome (CAIS), the best approach is to provide a full explanation to the patient. Because the patient is not able to respond to the testosterone or other androgens that the body produces but does respond to estrogen, the patient has imprinted as a female and will likely choose to live as a female, but this decision must be made by the patient.

129. B: When screening an older adult for depression with the Geriatric Depression Scale, short form (GDS-SF) with 15 questions, the minimal score that indicates possible depression is 6 (>5). Patients answer "yes/no" to questions about their satisfaction with life, feelings, memory problems, and general situation, with "yes" answers indicating depression. Patients who score greater than 5 should be further evaluated. A score greater than 10 almost always indicates depression. The short form requires about 5 to 7 minutes to complete. A long form with 30 questions is also available, although the short form is more commonly used for screening.

130. D: During registration, a new patient must sign an assignment of benefits form so that the provider can bill the insurance companies and receive reimbursement for claims directly. If there is no assignment of benefits, then the patient files the claim with the insurance company rather than the provider. This is sometimes the case if a patient is seeing a healthcare provider that is not in his/her network and doesn't, therefore, bill the insurance for care provided.

131. A: Orthopnea, frequent yawning, and sighing may indicate increased respiratory compromise in a person with myasthenia gravis (MG), so a complete respiratory assessment is warranted, including pulmonary function tests and pulse oximetry. The acetylcholine receptor (AChR) antibody titer is used to diagnose autoimmune MG. Repetitive nerve stimulation assesses neuromuscular transmission. The ice pack test consists of applying an ice pack to ptosis for 2 minutes and then evaluating the ptosis. Improvement is positive for MG.

132. C: Asking the patient to count backward from 20 to 1 can help identify an attention deficit. Other signs of delirium include language and memory disturbance, disorientation, confusion, audiovisual hallucinations, and sleep disturbance. Delirium, different from disorders with similar symptoms, is fluctuating. Delirium may result from drugs, infection, hypoxia, trauma, dementia, depression, vision and hearing loss, surgery, alcoholism, untreated pain, fluid/electrolyte imbalance, and malnutrition. Treatment includes providing a sitter to ensure safety and decreasing dosages of hypnotics and psychotropics. Protocols for side rails and restraints must be followed,

and restraints are used as a last resort. Medications to reduce symptoms include trazodone, lorazepam, and haloperidol.

133. C: The total nutrient admixture (TNA) should be discarded if there is "cracking" of the lipid emulsion and the oil separates into a layer. With TNA, all the components of parenteral nutrition and lipids are admixed together in one container to create a 3-in-1 formula. Components of parenteral nutrition generally include proteins, carbohydrates, fats, electrolytes, vitamins, sterile water, and trace vitamins. Whereas most postoperative patients need 1500 calories per day to prevent protein breakdown, those patients with fever, burns, major surgery, trauma, or hypermetabolic disease will require additional calories.

134. D: Autonomy is the ethical principle that the individual has the right to make decisions about his/her own care. The AGACNP must keep patients fully informed so they can exercise autonomy in informed decision making. Beneficence is an ethical principle that involves performing actions that are for the purpose of benefiting another person. Nonmaleficence is an ethical principle that means healthcare workers should provide care in a manner that does not cause direct intentional harm to the patient. Justice is the ethical principle that relates to the distribution of the limited resources of healthcare benefits to the members of society.

135. A: If a 24-year-old patient diagnosed with type 1 diabetes mellitus with a glucose level of 468 mg/dL (26 mmol/L), polyuria, polydipsia, and weight loss has stabilized since starting insulin injections and now appears to be able to manage the diabetes with very little insulin, the AGACNP should suspect that the patient's insulin needs will increase again. Symptoms of diabetes usually don't occur until about destruction of 90% of the pancreatic islet. Once stabilized, the patient often undergoes a "honeymoon" period when the remaining cells seem to produce enough insulin, but the same process of cell destruction and increased blood glucose will continue.

136. C: Adolescents respond well to a combination of a selective serotonin reuptake inhibitor (SSRI) and cognitive behavioral therapy (CBT) for the treatment of depression, but SSRI use in adolescents has been associated with increased suicidal ideation, so the girl must be carefully monitored and assessed. She and her family should be educated about this possible effect and warning signs of suicidal ideation. In some cases, adolescents may be asked to sign a no-suicide contract that clearly outlines the steps to take in the event that they feel suicidal.

137. D: "I'd like to hear how you feel" is an example of therapeutic communication that allows a patient to explore a topic. Nontherapeutic communication includes the following:

- Meaningless clichés: "Don't worry. Everything will be fine." "Isn't it a nice day?"
- Providing advice: "You should..." or "The best thing to do is...." It's better when patients ask for advice to provide facts and encourage the patient to reach a decision.
- Asking for explanations of behavior that is not directly related to patient care and requires analysis and explanation of feelings: "Why are you upset?"

138. D: The best solution is a referral to a home health agency to provide in-home care because this ensures that the woman will receive skilled nursing care and be able to stay at home and supervise her granddaughter. A 12-year-old child is too young for the responsibility for wound care. The patient's dependence on public transportation and difficulty walking preclude outpatient care. Home health care is a more cost-effective solution than transferring the patient to an extended care facility, which would leave the granddaughter without care. Medicare will not pay for extended hospital care for healing wounds.

139. C: If a patient has a long leg cast and requires assessment to ensure that the cast is not restrictive, the 5 P's assessment include the following:

The 5 P's of neurovascular assessment	
Pain	Determine the site, extent, duration, changes.
Pallor	Evaluate overall color and color distal to injuries, casts. Pallor or cyanosis indicates impaired circulation or venous stasis.
Pulselessness	Assess distal pulses and compare to other pulses. A weak or absent pulse may indicate impaired circulation.
Paresthesia	Assess for tingling, numbness, or other abnormal sensations because these many indicate nerve damage or compartment syndrome.
Paralysis	Assess for motion distal and proximal to cast because the inability to move may also indicate nerve damage or compartment syndrome.

140. A: Glycopyrrolate or atropine subcutaneously (subQ) has a rapid onset of action (about 1 minute). Glycopyrrolate provides stronger action. Morphine sulfate may reduce respiratory distress but does not generally affect death rattles. The hyoscine hydrobromide (scopolamine) transdermal patch has a slow onset of action (about 12 hours), so it is best used for long-term treatment. Oropharyngeal suctioning may relieve rattles originating in the oropharynx but is ineffective for pooling of fluids in the bronchi.

141. D: The following symptoms are consistent with pacemaker syndrome:

Mild	Pulsations evident in the neck and abdomen. Cardiac palpitations. Headache and feeling of anxiety. General malaise and unexplained weakness. Pain or "fullness" in jaw, chest.
Moderate	Increasing dyspnea on exertion with accompanying orthopnea. Dizziness, vertigo, increasing confusion. Feeling of choking.
Severe	Increasing pulmonary edema with dyspnea even at rest and crackling rales. Syncope. Heart failure.

142. A: A cost-benefit analysis uses the average cost of a problem (such as wound infections) and the cost of intervention to demonstrate savings. For example, if a surgical unit averaged 10 surgical site infections annually at an additional average cost of $27,000 each, the total annual cost would be $270,000. If the total cost for interventions, (new staff person, benefits, education, and software) totals $92,000, and the goal is to reduce infections by 50% (5 × $27,000 for a total projected savings of $135,000), the cost benefit is demonstrated by subtracting the proposed savings from the intervention costs ($135,000–$92,000) for a savings of $43,000 annually.

143. D: Root cause analysis is a retrospective attempt to determine the cause of an event. Regression analysis compares the relationship between two variables to determine if the relationship correlates. The t-test is used to analyze data to determine if there is a statistically significant difference in the means of two groups. The t-test looks at two sets of things that are similar, such as exercise in women older than 65 with cancer and without cancer. The tracer methodology is a method that looks at the continuum of care a patient receives from admission to post discharge.

144. D: Active pulmonary tuberculosis (TB) is characterized by night sweats, cough, and low-grade fever. Cough usually persists for 3 weeks or longer and may be nonproductive or mucopurulent. As TB progresses, hemoptysis may occur. Night sweats are frequent and pronounced. Patients also have fatigue, weight loss, and anorexia. Patients may have chest pain and pain on coughing. Extrapulmonary manifestations may result in meningitis, scrofula of the neck, TB pleurisy, miliary TB, Pott's disease (bones and spine), and urogenital TB.

145. A: If, as leader of an interdisciplinary team, the AGACNP notes that one team member who has worked on the unit for more than 20 years frequently criticizes younger and less experienced nurses, the best initial approach to resolve this is to ask the experienced nurse to serve as a mentor. This shows recognition of the nurse's skills and may help to alleviate some anxiety the nurse may have about being displaced by younger nurses.

146. B: The purpose of the Quality and Safety Education for Nurses (QSEN) initiatives is to ensure that quality and safety competencies are incorporated into the education of nurses. The three elements that QSEN focuses on are (1) knowledge, (2) skills, and (3) attitudes (KSA). Nurses are encouraged to review standards and nursing practice and to find better ways to deliver safe and effective care. QSEN includes six components: patient-centered care, teamwork and collaboration, evidence-based practice, safety, quality improvement, and informatics.

147. C: If a patient is prescribed five different medications, the chance of drug interactions because of polypharmacy is approximately 50%. Although the risk for drug interactions is only 6% if a patient takes two drugs, the more drugs a patient takes, the more the risk increases. Those patients taking eight drugs have about a 100% chance of drug interactions. For this reason, it's important to carry out drug reconciliation at each visit and to carefully consider previous prescriptions when ordering new drugs.

148. D: If a 36-year-old woman comes to the emergency department complaining of vaginal discharge that started two days prior to the expected onset of menstruation, the findings consistent with vaginal candidiasis include severe vaginal and vulvar itching and thick, white, adherent (cottage-cheese-appearing) discharge. Candidiasis is common shortly before menstruation because the vaginal pH falls. Onset is usually rapid. Patients who are immunocompromised are at increased risk of developing vaginal candidiasis. Treatment includes oral fluconazole or topical regimens (including clotrimazole and miconazole).

149. B: The patient's response is probably culturally different from what the nurse expects. Nurses and doctors are viewed with respect, so traditional Asian families may expect the nurse to remain authoritative and to give directions and may not question authority. The nurse should ensure that Asian patients understand by having them review material or give demonstrations and should provide explanations clearly, anticipating questions that the family might not articulate. Disagreeing is considered impolite. "Yes" may only mean that the person is heard, not that there is agreement with the person; therefore, patients and their families may indicate that they understand even when they clearly do not to avoid offending the nurse.

150. A: Cushing's triad (hypertension, bradycardia, and widening pulse pressure) in patients with increased intracranial pressure from a traumatic brain injury may be a sign of brain herniation. Cushing's triad is always an indication of very poor prognosis and may result from severe hemorrhage or a large-space-occupying tumor. Brain (or cerebral) herniation means that the brain tissue shifts from its normal position, so various parts of the brain may be involved, and the shift can be upward, downward, or lateral.

151. B: If 15 hours after a patient was involved in an automobile accident the patient presents in the emergency department with abdominal discomfort and a positive Cullen's sign (bruising about the umbilicus), the AGACNP should suspect retroperitoneal bleeding or hemoperitoneum. This sign is usually not evident for about 12 hours. Other indications include a positive Grey Turner's sign (bruising over the flank). The patient may also have hematuria and hemodynamic instability.

152. D: The first step in diagnosing an acid-base disturbance is to evaluate the pH, using 7.4 as the starting point (the normal range is from 7.35 to 7.45). If the pH is less than 7.4, it is becoming more acidotic, and if the pH is greater than 7.5, it is becoming more alkalotic. Next, the pCO_2 is evaluated because high levels indicate acidosis and low levels indicate alkalosis. Then the HCO_3 is evaluated, with high levels indicating alkalosis and low levels indicating acidosis. Next, evaluate the pH in relation to CO_2 and HCO_3 to determine respiratory or metabolic alkalosis or acidosis. Last, evaluate for compensation.

153. A: The PQRST method to assess chest pain is described as follows:

- P—Precipitating events: Exercise, emotions, rest, eating.
- Q—Quality of pain/discomfort: Dull, sharp, aching, restricting, crushing, suffocating.
- R—Radiation of pain: upper chest, mid-chest, neck, shoulders, arms, back.
- S—Severity of pain: Scale of 1–10.
- T—Timing: Time of onset, changes since onset, history of previous episodes.

Chest pain indicates risk of heart attack, and many patients do not experience symptoms such as chest pain until their coronary arteries are 70% occluded, even though a 50% occlusion is significant in terms of morbidity/mortality.

154. C: Following gastric bypass surgery that includes removal of the pyloric valve, dumping syndrome is often precipitated by high-sugar (carbohydrate) foods, such as candy, desserts, pasta, and fruit. Food and gastric juices move rapidly from the stomach into the intestines because the valve is missing. Symptoms usually occur within 30 minutes of ingestion and include nausea, vomiting, abdominal pain/cramping, distension, diarrhea, tachycardia, and dizziness. Similar symptoms may occur 1 to 3 hours after eating, in addition to diaphoresis, weakness, fatigue, tremors, anxiety, and mental confusion. Increased insulin levels may cause hypoglycemia.

155. B: When examining a patient's breasts for masses, the AGACNP is aware that the most common site for breast cancer is the upper lateral quadrant of the breast.

Incidence by area of the breast:

- Upper medial quadrant: 15%.
- Upper lateral quadrant: 55%.
- Lower medial quadrant: 5%.
- Lower lateral quadrant: 10%.
- Areola/Nipple: 15%.

Breast abnormalities that may indicate breast cancer include masses, skin dimpling, changes in texture or color of the skin, change in nipple appearance, and clear or sanguineous discharge from the nipple.

156. D: About 70% of cervical cancer cases are linked to a history of human papilloma virus (HPV), even though many people with HPV infection are asymptomatic. Recent studies indicate that approximately 69% of Americans have been infected with HPV. The strains that are most likely to

cause cancer are HPV-16 and HPV-18. HPV vaccinations are available and are recommended for children at ages 11 or 12, but if someone is not vaccinated as a child, the vaccinations are recommended for females through age 26 and males through age 21 to 26, depending on risk factors.

157. A: If the AGACNP overhears a nurse complain that if the hospital treats an uninsured homeless patient, it will be overwhelmed with many more homeless patients and go bankrupt, the type of logical fallacy this represents is the slippery slope. The slippery slope is the assumption that one action (treating the uninsured homeless patient) will lead to a chain of events (many more homeless patients) that culminate in disaster (bankruptcy).

158. C: If a patient who has taken opioids for pain for a prolonged period complains that the drugs are less effective, the adaptive state in which the effects of the drugs diminish over time is opioid tolerance. As patients develop tolerance, they may need higher doses of medication to achieve the same results, but this can lead to increasing physical and psychological dependence, so the patient may need to be referred to a pain specialist to learn alternate means of controlling pain.

159. B: If a patient with a head injury has a slightly elevated intracranial pressure (ICP) but develops a high fever, the AGACNP expects the fever to increase both the ICP and the cerebral perfusion pressure (CPP) because the fever increases the metabolic rate and causes vasodilation. Fever is common after brain injury and may be directly related to the neurologic injury because other causes are often not found. Fever elevation of even 1°C must be treated aggressively with acetaminophen, cooling blankets, and cold infusions if necessary.

160. D: Restrictive cardiomyopathy is a heart condition in which stiffened heart muscles cannot contract adequately. Although the ability to contract and the thickness of the myocardial wall remains normal, the heart is unable to relax enough to fill the ventricles with blood, so the blood backs up into the atria, resulting in increased peripheral and pulmonary edema. Fainting is often the first symptom, and sudden cardiac arrest may occur. Restrictive cardiomyopathy is usually more severe with childhood onset.

161. A: The Centers for Disease Control and Prevention (CDC) recommends that the following people should be screened for hepatitis C:

- People born from 1945 through 1965.
- People with medical conditions such as HIV/AIDS and chronic liver disease.
- People who have ever injected drugs or shared needles even once.
- People whose liver tests are abnormal.
- People who received donated organs or blood prior to 1992.
- Healthcare workers who experienced exposure to blood (needlestick or other injury).
- All patients receiving hemodialysis.
- All people born to a mother infected with hepatitis C.

Note: People often do not show symptoms until the disease is advanced.

162. D: The pH of urine usually ranges from 4.5 to 8 (average 5 to 6). Some medications may make urine more acidic (<7 pH), such as Mandelamine and vitamin C, and some foods, such as cranberries. If the urine is alkaline (>7 pH), this may indicate bacteriuria, urinary tract infections, as well as kidney and respiratory diseases. Urine may appear cloudy with infection, and bacteria in the urine may give the urine a foul odor. Culture and sensitivity is done to identify infective agents.

163. A: If a patient is on the National Dysphagia Diet 1 (NND1) (Dysphagia—pureed) diet, foods that would be excluded include scrambled eggs, peanut butter, gelatin, yogurt with fruit (unless it is smooth and completely blended), and cottage cheese. The patient is allowed food with no lumps with the consistency of smooth pudding. These foods can include pureed meats, fruits, vegetables, soups, smooth mashed potatoes, ice cream, and puddings. Foods must be pureed with sufficient broth/liquid so they don't adhere to the patient's mouth.

164. B: If a patient is unable to take four steps or bear weight on an injured knee, this likely indicates the need for an X-ray to evaluate a probable fracture. Other indications include age over 55, isolated tenderness of the patella, and tenderness at the head of the fibula. With a fractured knee, the patient is not able to flex the knee to 90°. Fractures should be suspected with open wounds or major soft-tissue trauma.

165. C: If a patient with rheumatoid arthritis (RA) complains of dry eyes, dry mouth, dry lips, and increasing dysphagia, the extra-articular manifestation of RA that the AGACNP should suspect is Sjogren's syndrome. This is an autoimmune disorder occurring in 10 to 15% of patients with RA. Antibodies attack primarily the lacrimal and salivary glands, although in some cases other glands, such as those lining the breathing passages and the vagina, may also be involved.

166. A: Nonalcoholic fatty liver disease occurs when fat is deposited in the liver and can eventually lead to scarring and cirrhosis. The most common risk factors are diabetes mellitus type 2, obesity, insulin resistance, and metabolic syndrome. The first-line treatment is to encourage the patient to gradually lose 10% or more of his or her body weight, but some improvement may be realized with a 3% to 5% loss. The patient should be counseled in healthy eating and exercise habits.

167. C: If the AGACNP is sexually harassed by a member of the medical staff in an episode witnessed by three coworkers, but the coworkers say they do not want to be involved when the AGACNP documents the harassment in an incident report, the most appropriate action is to file the incident report and list witnesses. Sexual harassment is illegal, and, should the case go to court, coworkers may not be willing to commit perjury even though they were willing to overlook the abuse.

168. B: If a 38-year-old male patient comes to the emergency department with severe left flank pain from a kidney stone, the priority treatment should be to administer analgesia. An alpha-blocker, such as tamsulosin, may also be administered to help to relax the distal ureter and promote passage of the stone. Patients who are to undergo surgical removal are kept on a nothing-by-mouth (NPO) status until after the procedure; otherwise, patients are advised to increase hydration to 3 to 4 L daily.

169. D: Patients with a history of alcoholism often have poor quality sleep and restlessness for weeks or years even after stopping drinking. With alcohol, sedation occurs early with acute intoxication but is later replaced with increased wakefulness and restlessness. Excessive alcohol may also worsen symptoms of obstructive sleep apnea or central sleep apnea. In fact, people with no signs of sleep apnea may exhibit episodes of obstructive sleep apnea after heavy drinking because breathing is more shallow and slower and the muscles of the throat are relaxed.

170. C: Hydrotherapy is contraindicated for venous ulcers because the warm water causes vasodilation, which may worsen the wound condition. Wounds that result from arterial insufficiency usually don't benefit from hydrotherapy. Hydrotherapy may be used with diabetic ulcers, but care must be taken to monitor the temperature carefully because the patient may be insensitive to heat because of neuropathy. Hydrotherapy is most often used to treat large wounds,

such as burns, but cross-contamination may occur if the equipment is not thoroughly disinfected. The water temperature should be 37°C.

171. A: Silver sulfadiazine (2%–7%) is frequently used to treat burns to promote healing and prevent infection with Gram-positive organisms, such as *Staphylococcus aureus,* methicillin-resistant *Staphylococcus aureus* (MRSA), *Streptococcus,* and *Pseudomonas.* Cadexomer iodine contains beads that swell in contact with exudate, releasing iodine in the wound. Iodine is effective against numerous bacteria, viruses, and fungi. Polymyxin B is used for small cuts and wounds to protect against Gram-positive organisms. Mupirocin is also effective against Gram-positive organisms and is used to treat skin infections and nasal colonization.

172. B: The AGACNP should advise using hydrogel dressings for a full-thickness necrotic wound with a small amount of exudate. Hydrogel dressings can be used in infected and necrotic wounds if they are dry or if the exudate is minimal. Hydrogel comes in a number of different forms: paste, sheets, and packing strips. The dressings are applied directly to the wound to create moisture and autolysis. Hydrogel dressings are covered with a secondary dressing.

173. D: Because of the high incidence of comorbidity, a patient who has been diagnosed with Addison's disease (primary adrenal insufficiency) should be screened for celiac disease, and the opposite is also true. These two disorders have been linked, suggesting that they may share genetic traits, especially in patients who have autoimmune polyendocrine syndrome, a condition in which Addison's disease is associated with thyroid disease. People with celiac disease are intolerant to gluten and must maintain a gluten-free diet to control symptoms.

174. C: If a patient is hospitalized with Guillain-Barré syndrome, the treatment of choice is plasmapheresis or intravenous immunoglobulin therapy (high-dose IVIg). There is no cure, but these treatments do relieve symptoms and accelerate recovery. IVIg is used most frequently, but the results are similar, and there is no advantage to using both treatments. Other treatments are supportive and may include intubation and ventilation if the patient develops respiratory failure. Most patients who are hospitalized with GBS have acute respiratory distress syndrome.

175. A: Patients with long-term urinary catheters are at high risk of developing resistant infections because of the development of biofilms in the bladder. *Staphylococcus aureus* is particularly dangerous because it is virulent and has the ability to form biofilms, in which cells adhere to tissue and accumulate in large clusters that secrete a polysaccharide substance that protects the cells from antibiotics. Biofilms are very hard to treat because the bacteria become resistant and disperse. Urinary catheters should be used only if absolutely necessary and for the shortest possible period.

176. D: Evolving changes related to melanomas are listed as follows:

The ABCDEs of melanomas
Asymmetry.
Borders uneven, scalloped, or notched.
Color variations within a mole.
Diameter is usually larger than 1/4 inch (6 mm).
Evolving changes in size, shape, color, or appearance.

Melanomas can occur anywhere on the body but are most common on the torso, head, and neck of males and the legs of females. People with dark skin may develop melanoma on the nailbeds, palms, and soles of the feet.

177. B: Patients who have sickle cell disease receive hydroxyurea to decrease sickling of red blood cells. It is prescribed for adults who experience three or more vaso-occlusive crises a year. Hydroxyurea stimulates production of fetal hemoglobin (because this form of hemoglobin reduces sickling) and reduces the production of reticulocytes and neutrophils, so the white blood cell (WBC) count is lower. High WBC counts are associated with increased morbidity. Hydroxyurea may increase the risk of infection.

178. A: The AGACNP should warn a patient who is prescribed varenicline (Chantix) for nicotine dependence to be alert for psychiatric symptoms and suicidal ideation. Adverse effects may include depression, aggressive behavior, psychosis, mania, and anxiety. The patient may experience homicidal and suicidal ideation, so family members should be advised to be on alert for psychiatric symptoms. Patients should be closely monitored while on varenicline, which reduces withdrawal symptoms associated with smoking cessation.

179. C: As part of stroke rehabilitation, the primary purpose of functional electrical stimulation devices is to improve the patient's functional ability. Electrodes are placed on the skin to stimulate the nerves and cause the muscle to contract. Some devices, such as those produced by Bioness for the arm and leg, are wireless and are easily applied. Most devices have different settings so they can be adjusted for various types of repetitive exercises, such as grasping.

180. D: If a patient on hemodialysis has an arteriovenous fistula (AVF) in the right forearm and requires a blood draw, the blood should be drawn from the left arm. The extremity with the AVF or other hemodialysis vascular device should never be used for venipuncture, IV fluids, or blood pressure because it's important to maintain the integrity of the vascular access. Patients often have extensive scarring of the blood vessels, so venipuncture can be challenging.

181. A: If a patient complains of sudden-onset "tearing" chest pain associated with severe back pain, the AGACNP should suspect that the origin of the pain is aortic dissection. Aortic dissection involves a tear in the aortic wall that allows blood to seep between the layers, leading to rupture. Patients may present with various types of symptoms depending on the site of the dissection and the degree. If the aortic dissection occurs in the abdominal aorta, then the pain is in the abdominal area.

182. C: If an 80-year-old patient with peripheral arterial disease states he has severe pain in the dorsum and toes of the right foot and toes when lying in bed at night, but the pain is relieved somewhat when he stands up, these symptoms indicate possible critical limb ischemia. When lying flat, the blood pressure drops and the arteries may be almost completely occluded, but the pressure of gravity may allow some circulation (relieving pain) when the patient is standing. Surgical revascularization is usually necessary to avoid amputation.

183. B: If a patient with multiple sclerosis (MS) has shown steady progression of the disease since diagnosis but has periodic episodes of acute exacerbations and remissions, this type of MS is classified as progressive relapsing. This type affects only about 5% of patients with MS. Each exacerbation tends to be progressively more severe than the previous one, so there is a steady progression of symptoms. Additionally, the patient tends to deteriorate to some degree between relapses.

184. D: If a patient asks the AGACNP about the feasibility of traveling to a high elevation (higher than 13,000 feet) in the mountains of Colorado to stay with family members after discharge from the hospital, the condition that would preclude such travel is sickle cell disease. The hypoxemia at high altitude, even above 2000 m, can precipitate an occlusive crisis or splenic crisis. Patients who must travel to a higher elevation may require oxygen during travel.

185. A: If a patient who has been intubated for 3 days is now breathing independently and is to begin oral fluids, the initial action should be to carry out a bedside swallowing test. A patient who has been intubated, especially for more than 48 hours, has an increased risk of pharyngeal dysfunction and dysphagia. The patient should be carefully observed while drinking 50 mL of water to determine if he or she chokes, coughs, or aspirates (often resulting in decreased oxygen saturation).

186. C: If a patient has a proximal small-bowel obstruction with abdominal pain and distension, the AGACNP also likely documents rapid onset of nausea and projective vomiting of bile emesis. If the obstruction is in the distal small intestine, then the nausea usually develops more slowly and the emesis tends to be orange-brown in color and with a fecal odor or fecal residue. If the obstruction results from strangulation, then emergent surgical repair is necessary, but many cases resolve with conservative treatment (IV fluids, NG tube).

187. B: Although maggots are unpleasant at best, their presence in an open venous stasis ulcer on the lower leg of a homeless patient likely helped to debride the ulcer. In fact, medical maggots are FDA-approved for wound debridement, although they are infrequently used because most people find them repulsive. Maggots need a moist environment to work most effectively, so after application of maggots to a wound, saline soaks are applied and remoistened frequently. There is some risk of infection from maggots.

188. D: If the AGACNP asks the patient stick out the tongue and examines the thrust for symmetry and then asks the patient to say "light, tight, dynamite," the cranial nerve that the AGACNP is evaluating is cranial nerve XII, the hypoglossal nerve. Abnormalities include atrophy of the tongue tissue, fasciculations, and deviation to the side of the nerve injury or paralysis.

189. B: If one parent carries the dominant mutation for Huntington's disease, an autosomal dominant disorder, and the other does not, each child has a 50% chance of having the disease. There is no carrier state without the disease. Because there is no cure for the disease, testing of children is not advised. They should be allowed as adults to decide whether or not they want genetic testing.

N = normal gene. **D** = dominant mutated gene.

	N	**D**
N	N N	N D disease
N	N N	N D disease

190. A: Negative symptoms of schizophrenia include flat affect, decreased emotional range, social isolation, poverty of speech, lack of interest, and lack of drive. Positive symptoms include delusions, hallucinations, disorganized or catatonic behavior, and disorganized speech. Patients with schizophrenia are usually oriented to person, place, and time, but their behavior may range widely. Some patients may exhibit unusual or atypical behavior, such as hoarding and water intoxication. Some may exhibit motor abnormalities, such as posturing or ritualistic behaviors.

191. C: The standard triple therapy for *Helicobacter pylori*-associated peptic ulcer disease includes a proton pump inhibitor two times a day (BID), clarithromycin 500 mg BID, and amoxicillin 1 g BID. Metronidazole 500 mg BID may be substituted for amoxicillin for those with penicillin allergy. Treatment is usually continued for 10 to 14 days. Using two antibiotics is especially important

because of the increasing incidence of resistant strains. The standard triple therapy is most commonly used, but a standard quadruple therapy and sequential quadruple therapy may also be considered.

192. B: Immigrants from Mexico are most at risk of having Chagas disease, which is frequently undiagnosed because of unfamiliarity with the disease. The disease is spread when a triatomine ("assassin" or "kissing") bug that is infected with *Trypanosoma cruzi* infects a human through feces deposited near a bite, allowing parasites in the feces to enter the body. Only about 1% of those infected show acute flu-like symptoms. Some may develop myocarditis, hepatomegaly, and splenomegaly. Chronic disease is characterized by cardiac disease, megaesophagus, and megacolon.

193. B: Symptoms that are common to patients with a tumor in the cerebellum include lack of coordination and balance. Patients may first notice ataxia and incoordination of the muscles before other symptoms. Because of increased intracranial pressure, patients may experience nausea and vomiting, especially in the morning and at night, as well as headache. Patients may experience increasing fatigue and lethargy. Diagnosis of a brain tumor is confirmed with neurological exam and magnetic resonance imaging (MRI).

194. A: Following a bout of West Nile fever, the symptom that is likely to persist for the longest period is fatigue, usually up to a month or longer. West Nile fever occurs in about 20% of those infected and lasts for up to 6 days. Onset is usually sudden with fever, nausea, vomiting, muscle aches, and enlarged lymph glands. A maculopapular rash on the trunk develops 3 to 7 days after onset of symptoms. West Nile-associated encephalitis and/or meningitis may also occur with severe neurological symptoms, including flaccid paralysis.

195. D: If a patient has returned home from a trip to Africa with symptoms of uncomplicated malaria, the stages would include the following:

- Cold stage: Chills, shivering.
- Hot stage: Fever (up to 41°C), headaches, flushed skin, vomiting, seizures.
- Sweating stage: Diaphoresis and then rapid return to normal temperature, weakness.

These symptoms may not be obvious at the onset of the disease but usually develop over the next 6 to 10 hours and may not appear in an exact rotation. Some patients may develop muscle aches and diarrhea as well.

196. A: Medications that can cause an increased risk of osteoporosis include corticosteroids. Doses greater than 2.5 mg per day of oral prednisone or equivalent increase risk. Some anticonvulsants, excessive thyroid hormones, chemotherapy used for the treatment of cancer such as methotrexate, antacids that contain aluminum hydroxide, cyclosporine, and heparin all increase the risk of developing osteoporosis. Some chronic diseases also increase the risk of osteoporosis, including rheumatoid arthritis, hyperthyroidism, Cushing's syndrome, Addison's disease, and hyperparathyroidism.

197. C: If a patient is hospitalized with heat exhaustion, 50% of the total water depletion should be replaced within the first 3 to 6 hours with the remaining replaced over the next 6 to 9 hours. For mild cases, oral rehydration with 0.1% isotonic sodium chloride solution should be given at the rate of 4 ounces every 15 to 20 minutes, but IV fluids will be needed for more severe cases. Water depletion is most common in elderly patients or with those who are physically active (such as runners) in hot weather but are not drinking enough water.

198. A: If a patient experiencing an acute episode of asthma is anxious, sitting in the tripod position with audible wheezing resulting from an upper airway obstruction with a peak flow of 65% of normal and oxygen saturation of 92%, the initial treatment should be the rescue protocol that generally begins with an inhaled short-acting beta-2 agonist, such as albuterol (Proventil HFA), to relax the smooth muscles. An anticholinergic, such as ipratropium bromide (Atrovent HFA), may also be given to relieve bronchospasm. If there is no improvement within 10 minutes, then a low-dose inhaled corticosteroid may be provided.

199. A: Angiotensin-converting enzyme (ACE) inhibitors and angiotensin II receptor blockers (ARBs) are less effective for treating hypertension in African-American patients, so treatment is often initiated with a diuretic or a diuretic combined with a calcium channel blocker. African-American patients are at increased risk for hypertension and diseases associated with hypertension, such as diabetes mellitus, but they tend to respond differently than Caucasians to standard treatments. The reason for this is not clear, but it may have a genetic component.

200. C: Timed up and go (TUG): The patient stands from a chair with armrests, walks 3 meters, and then turns and sits back down. Those patients requiring ≥14 seconds are at risk for falls (normal is 7–10 seconds). During assessment, the patient should be carefully observed for gait abnormalities, including unsteadiness, uneven weight distribution, abnormal position of limbs, and type of gait. Gait assessment also includes the following:

- Gait speed in 5 meters with slow gait (<0.6 m/second) predictive of functional limitations.
- Performance-oriented mobility assessment (POMA) tests mobility and gait under different conditions.

Thank You

We at Mometrix would like to extend our heartfelt thanks to you, our friend and patron, for allowing us to play a part in your journey. It is a privilege to serve people from all walks of life who are unified in their commitment to building the best future they can for themselves.

The preparation you devote to these important testing milestones may be the most valuable educational opportunity you have for making a real difference in your life. We encourage you to put your heart into it—that feeling of succeeding, overcoming, and yes, conquering will be well worth the hours you've invested.

We want to hear your story, your struggles and your successes, and if you see any opportunities for us to improve our materials so we can help others even more effectively in the future, please share that with us as well. **The team at Mometrix would be absolutely thrilled to hear from you!** So please, send us an email (support@mometrix.com) and let's stay in touch.

If you feel as though you need additional help, please check out the other resources we offer:

Study Guide: http://MometrixStudyGuides.com/NP

Flashcards: http://MometrixFlashcards.com/NP